Social Work Approaches in Health and Mental Health from Around the Globe

Social Work Approaches in Health and Mental Health from Around the Globe has been co-published simultaneously as *Social Work in Mental Health*, Volume 2, Numbers 2/3 2004.

Social Work Approaches in Health and Mental Health from Around the Globe

Anna Metteri, MSocSc
Teppo Kröger, PhD
Anneli Pohjola, PhD
Pirkko-Liisa Rauhala, PhD
Editors

Gary Rosenberg, PhD
Andrew Weissman, PhD
Series Editors

Social Work Approaches in Health and Mental Health from Around the Globe has been co-published simultaneously as *Social Work in Mental Health*, Volume 2, Numbers 2/3 2004.

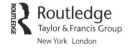

Routledge
Taylor & Francis Group
New York London

First published by

The Haworth Social Work Practice Press, 10 Alice Street, Binghamton, NY 13904-1580 USA

The Haworth Social Work Practice Press is an imprint of The Haworth Press, Inc., 10 Alice Street, Binghamton, NY 13904-1580 USA.

This edition published 2012 by Routledge

Routledge	Routledge
Taylor & Francis Group	Taylor & Francis Group
711 Third Avenue	2 Park Square, Milton Park
New York, NY 10017	Abingdon, Oxon OX14 4RN

Social Work Approaches in Health and Mental Health from Around the Globe has been co-published simultaneously as *Journal of Aggression, Maltreatment & Trauma*, Volume 2, Numbers 2/3 2004.

The development, preparation, and publication of this work has been undertaken with great care. However, the publisher, employees, editors, and agents of The Haworth Press and all imprints of The Haworth Press, Inc., including The Haworth Medical Press® and The Pharmaceutical Products Press®, are not responsible for any errors contained herein or for consequences that may ensue from use of materials or information contained in this work. Opinions expressed by the author(s) are not necessarily those of The Haworth Press, Inc.

Cover design by Jennifer Gaska

Library of Congress Cataloging-in-Publication Data

Social work approaches in health and mental health from around the globe / Anna Metteri . . . [et al.], editors.
    p. cm.
    "Co-published simultaneously as Social Work in mental health, volume 2, numbers 2/3, 2004."
    Includes bibliographical references and index.
    ISBN 0-7890-2512-4 (hbk. : alk. paper) – ISBN 0-7890-2513-2 (pbk: alk. paper)
    1. Medical social work. 2. Psychiatric social work. I. Metteri, Anna. II. Social work in mental health.
HV687 .S586 2004
362.1′042521–dc22
                                            2004003625

ABOUT THE EDITORS

Anna Metteri, MSocSc, is Associate Professor in Social Work at the Department of Social Policy and Social Work at the University of Tampere in Finland, where she is also finalizing her doctoral studies. She worked as a social work practitioner in health and mental health for 12 years before coming back to the University. She was nominated as Social Worker of the Year in 1993 in Finland. She was a member of the Nordic Committee of the Schools of Social Work from 1999-2003 and has been a member of the Executive Committee of the European Association of Schools of Social Work since 2003. She was chair of two international social work conferences held in Tampere: the 3rd International Conference on Social Work in Health and Mental Health "Visions from Around the Globe" (July 2001) and the 4th International Conference on Evaluation for Practice (July 2002). Both conferences were meeting places for practitioners and academics and Metteri was nominated as congress organizer for the year 2002 in Tampere. She was the leader and teacher in charge of six professional postgraduate programmes (from 1 to 3 years each) in social work in health and mental health and empowering social work at the University's Centre for Extension Studies from 1991-2001. Her current research and teaching interests include social work practice in health and mental health, interdisciplinary education in mental health, and the development of agency in social work. She has been in charge of several collaborative research projects together with practicing social workers and service users. She is the author of many scientific and professional publications, which include six edited books, one co-authored book, numerous journal articles, book chapters, and conference proceedings.

Teppo Kröger, PhD, is Lecturer of Social Work in the Department of Social Sciences and Philosophy at the University of Jyväskylä in Finland, and Docent of Social Work in the Department of Social Policy and Social Work at the University of Tampere in Finland. He is a member of the Nordic Committee of Schools of Social Work. He was a member of the local organizing committee of the 3rd International Conference on

Health and Mental Health in Tampere in July of 2001. He has lectured widely on issues connected to social care. In addition to his publications in Finnish, Dr. Kröger has published articles in English in the *Scandinavian Journal of Social Welfare,* the *Journal of Social Policy,* the *Nordic Journal of Social Work*, and in several edited books. In 2001, the European Commission published his book "Comparative Research on Social Care: The State of the Art." Recently, he has coordinated a large comparative research project on combining the use of formal and informal care with participation in paid employment, funded by the European Commission.

Anneli Pohjola, PhD, is Academy Researcher in the Academy of Finland and works at the University of Lapland in Rovaniemi, Finland, where she previously served as a lecturer and research in social work. She has worked for Finland's Ministry of Education as a project administrator for social work education. She is a member of an expert group in the EC Phare Consensus Program "Training of Social Workers in Lithuania" and is one of three experts called upon by the Estonian Higher Education Accreditation Centre to evaluate social work education in Estonia. At the national level, she has held many confidential posts at the ministry of Social Affairs and Health, such as a member of the research section of the Consultative Committe for Equality, a member of the Consultative Committee of Social Work, and a member of the management group of Networking Special Services.

Pirkko-Liisa Rauhala, PhD, is University Lecturer of Social Work at the University of Helsinki in Finland, and Visiting Professor of Social Policy and Social Work at the University of Tartu in Estonia. She is an expert member of the Welfare Research Financing Committee of the Nordic Council of Ministers and has served as a scientific advisor to the UNFPA/Expert Group on Population Ageing and Development. She is a member of the European Social Policy Research Group at the Europaeische Akademie in Germany and a member of the Finnish Literature Society.

Social Work Approaches in Health and Mental Health from Around the Globe

CONTENTS

Introduction

This volume is based on the material gathered in the Third International Conference on Social Work in Health and Mental Health held in Tampere, Finland, in 2001, under the umbrella theme "Visions from Around the Globe." The discussions and presentations in the conference have given birth to three separate works, each addressing questions under a theme of its own, ranging from the social work viewpoint on citizenship and clients, to social work methods and social work approaches. The focus of this volume is on different approaches and orientations of social work in health and mental health.

This collection of articles bring out the diversity of social work in health and mental health and its many interfaces. The aim of the Tampere conference was to bring those doing research and developing the discipline in the academy and those developing the practice and the discipline in the field to the same forum for discussions and debate. As a result, a number of new, creative, theoretical, and practical orientations were brought forward for more developed ways of analyzing work. The texts open up views that comprise "something old, something new, something borrowed and something blue," to quote an old saying, and this combination will strengthen the basis of our understanding of social work. In global discourse, social issues are shaped in new ways, and understanding of those issues is rebuilt at the same time. The articles emphasize the common global features of social work in health and mental health on the one hand, and the diversity of the work on the other.

This volume is thematically divided into four sections. In the first section the focus is on the development of social work expertise in health and mental

[Haworth co-indexing entry note]: "Introduction." Pohjula, Anneli et al. Co-published simultaneously in *Social Work in Mental Health* (The Haworth Social Work Practice Press, an imprint of The Haworth Press, Inc.) Vol. 2, No. 2/3, 2004, pp. 1-5; and: *Social Work Approaches in Health and Mental Health from Around the Globe* (ed: Metteri et al.) The Haworth Social Work Practice Press, an imprint of The Haworth Press, Inc., 2004, pp. 1-5. Single or multiple copies of this article are available for a fee from The Haworth Document Delivery Service [1-800-HAWORTH, 9:00 a.m. - 5:00 p.m. (EST). E-mail address: docdelivery@haworthpress.com].

http://www.haworthpress.com/web/SWMH
Digital Object Identifier: 10.1300/J200v2n02_01

health. The two articles in the first section span a century of social work history, from the origins of the social work in health care to the challenges of today. The first article discusses the pioneering work of Richard C. Cabot in early medical social work. The second article reports on the results of the empirical study into the composition of the expertise of today's social workers in mental health care.

What the articles in the second section share is the notion of social work in health and mental health as an agent of change in society that crosses borders, operates on many levels and across many dimensions. However, the topics of the three articles are very diverse. The first article analyzes social work in health theoretically, developing a new interpretation of a holistic ecological model. The second article describes the challenges faced by social work starting from scratch in a newly independent country and the role of practice teaching as part of social development. The third article raises the question of outcomes measurement in social work in its many dimensions.

The third section emphasizes the basic questions of community based care. It is through communities that the global and the local aspects of social work are merging together in a very interesting way. The viewpoints of the five articles include the role of the social worker in health and mental health care as the coordinator of community based work, finding new conceptual frameworks for work with marginalized groups, ways of understanding community work and its working principles, concern for the client-oriented perspective and various community based forms of care.

The articles in the fourth section deal with the dual divisions so often present in social work that challenge social workers in health and mental health to become aware of and choose their own positions in work practice. On the other hand, concern for human rights is a task that makes social workers in this field cross dual divisions. Working for human rights requires effort in all dimensions. The two articles in this section discuss these basic questions and bring clients into focus with their life situations and their conditions.

This collection of articles provides a valuable stepping stone towards understanding that the basis of social work in health and mental health is the same throughout the world despite differences between countries in terms of culture, social system, and history. There is a common foundation of terminology, values, and basic tasks that turns out to be essential for learning from the experiences and thinking of others in creative interaction. The texts cover a long period in the history of social work in health issues. Geographically and culturally the articles cover a wide range of viewpoints from the North to the South, from the East to the West. The focus of the articles varies from theoretical treatises to empirical research and analyses of practices. The articles approach the global dimension in a totally different way from the dominant economic discourse.

What appears to be one joint basis of globality in the articles is the emphasis on the integration of theory and practice characteristic of social work in health and mental health. It is based on the equal appreciation of different knowledge bases, according to which inquiring and theoretical thinking form an integral part of the practical work process, while in research the formation of knowledge is powered by practice. The different origins of knowledge do not mean that knowledge is from different levels, but different types of knowledge support one another. The processes in both research and practical work follow the same basic methodological logic: They include similar phases and produce information on questions under analysis. Appreciating both knowledge bases enables progress in social work so that writing traditions can be reformed, new methodological approaches can be created and different, also, alternative knowledge and theory can be formed.

Evidence-based social work is often referred to as a prerequisite for work development. Nevertheless, it is important to discuss knowledge-based, research-based, and value-based social work as well as experience-based practice. Without all of these it is difficult to fully realize the development of work quality, definition of best practices, assessment of work output, and outcomes measurement.

The second joint feature of globality that the articles display is the emergence of similar issues and themes, even though the writers come from different parts of the world. This illustrates the fact that social life is basically human and very organized. There are more similarities than differences between people. Understanding this basic truth is one of the challenges of social work in health and mental health while still seeing each person as a unique individual who attaches meanings to things and situations differently from others. This interface between the general human and the unique individual is connected to the principle that social workers do not solve problem situations on the basis of "how things should be."

Thirdly, joint globality is characterized in the texts by the fact that social work is carried out on many different levels. It is this particular feature that makes social work in health and mental health so challenging: It ranges from meeting the needs of individuals, families, and communities and operating on the level of villages and municipalities to influencing welfare-related decision-making on the regional and national level and understanding also global issues affecting everyday work. Social work action in health care is permeated by supra-cultural features and events on the one hand and an increasing discourse on locality and people's life context on the other. The tasks range from social development to helping individual people in their acute distress. These are aspects that show how closely the humanly universal and the humanly particular are intertwined in social work.

In its dual role, social work in health and mental health operates first on the individual level to help citizens and clients, and second, it strives to change people's life contexts and to develop service systems on the level of society. Simultaneously it attempts both to individualize the client and make working environments more humane and more social. Structural development, service, and a related concern for citizens' rights are quite challenging to combine as orientations for work. It is inevitable that social work as an agent of change and social equality is working in society like a stone in a shoe. The multiplicity of tasks social workers in health and mental health care are tackling gives rise to contradictory demands and a diversity of expectations, which are also discussed in the articles.

The fourth characteristic of joint globality in the viewpoints of the articles can be seen in the way social work in this field is described as a profession and research topic that deals with difficult issues. Even though the emphasis in work is placed on influencing societal decision-making and on engagement in preventive action, the majority of issues are related to human distress and suffering, social exclusion and marginalization. The innate difficulty of this work sets challenges not only for social workers in their coping with everyday work, but also for those responsible for developing methodological tools and strengthening the common knowledge base of the discipline. One of the great merits of the articles lies in the analysis of the multidimensional relationships and challenges pertaining to social work in health and mental health.

According to the articles, social work operates in multilevel practice activities, it exposes workers to complicated and difficult situations, it deals with emotions and intensive relationships, and to achieve success, it calls for strong commitment to the client. All this creates a great deal of challenge for social workers: They need a versatile knowledge base, different methodological tools, and a strong value base. The extensive range of work in this field means that workers face many contradictions involved in their work, they tolerate ambiguity and cross borders, which are analyzed in many of the articles.

Social work in health and mental health as a whole is characterized by the fact that it operates across the boundaries of dual divisions or dichotomies. Some of the articles point out distinct dichotomies that come up in everyday work, such as health vs. mental health, the official aid system vs. various forms of informal help, reason vs. emotion, support–protection vs. control–obligation, exclusion vs. inclusion, micro level vs. macro level. To be able to navigate diverse emphases and orientations, social workers and researchers need solid epistemological, practical, and theoretical expertise. It is not merely a question of choosing one's side in twofold challenges but of mastery of the conceptual, ideological, and methodological aspects of the operational field. Being aware of this multiplexity is a prerequisite for choosing one's own position and transcending dualisms.

One conscientious choice that is stressed in the articles is the client-oriented basis of social work in health and mental health. Even though the bottom-up principle, partnership, and people's participation are used as orientations, multidimensionality emerges as an essential part of work. It is a challenge for the workers to be aware of the social mechanisms that produce poor chances, lack of hope, or stigmas. It is equally important to see the clients in their own situations as well as to understand the problems that affect them, which in turn means that environmental factors and the complexity of the service system are also at play in work practice. Many articles describe community work building on this foundation. They point out how service systems are incomplete and need reforming, and how small-scale improvements can be used to create better service by involving people and their environment in the work.

Social work in health and mental health care is under organizational pressure because social work is carried out in institutions dominated by other disciplines and professions. At the same time, the field is more interdisciplinary than in social work in average. The characteristic social expertise of social work is expanded methodologically by adapting and including, also, biological, psychological, political, economic, and philosophical knowledge. The multidimensionality of knowledge and awareness is a challenge of practice.

Anneli Pohjola
Anna Metteri
Teppo Kröger
Pirkko-Liisa Rauhala

SOCIAL WORK EXPERTISE IN HEALTH AND MENTAL HEALTH

Individualization and Prevention: Richard C. Cabot and Early Medical Social Work

Paul H. Stuart

SUMMARY. In 1905, Massachusetts General Hospital initiated the first medical social work program in the United States. Based on the writings of its leaders, this paper presents the early history of medical social work in the United States. Inspired by developments in European health care that emphasized the community context of disease, medical social work pioneers saw a need to individualize the patient while also promoting public health measures in the community, improving the patient's environment to eliminate the causes of disease. In addition, since they served patients because of their diseases rather than their poverty, medical social workers were among the first to provide social work ser-

Paul H. Stuart, PhD, is affiliated with the School of Social Work, University of Alabama, Box 870314, Tuscaloosa, AL 35487-0314 (E-mail: pstuart@sw.ua.edu).

[Haworth co-indexing entry note]: "Individualization and Prevention: Richard C. Cabot and Early Medical Social Work." Stuart, Paul H. Co-published simultaneously in *Social Work in Mental Health* (The Haworth Social Work Practice Press, an imprint of The Haworth Press, Inc.) Vol. 2, No. 2/3, 2004, pp. 7-20; and: *Social Work Approaches in Health and Mental Health from Around the Globe* (ed: Metteri et al.) The Haworth Social Work Practice Press, an imprint of The Haworth Press, Inc., 2004, pp. 7-20. Single or multiple copies of this article are available for a fee from The Haworth Document Delivery Service [1-800-HAWORTH, 9:00 a.m. - 5:00 p.m. (EST). E-mail address: docdelivery@haworthpress.com].

7

vices to the non-poor. In spite of their emphasis on environmental change, many of early medical social work leaders had an anti-institutional bias; they were suspicious of large-scale solutions for what they saw as fundamentally individual problems. Consequently, methods for promoting individual adaptation developed more rapidly than methods for promoting environmental change. Ironically, the medicalization of social problems in contemporary times has resulted in a focus on individual pathology rather than social and lifestyle causation in health, even as the rising cost and complexity of the system challenges health care consumers in the United States. Reaffirming the environmental emphasis of medical social work pioneers provides a way for today's health care social workers to incorporate environmental modification into their practice and promote the health of all citizens. *[Article copies available for a fee from The Haworth Document Delivery Service: 1-800-HAWORTH. E-mail address: <docdelivery@haworthpress.com> Website: <http:// www.HaworthPress.com> © 2004 by The Haworth Press, Inc. All rights reserved.]*

KEYWORDS. Richard C. Cabot, efficiency, history, individualization, Massachusetts General Hospital, prevention, progressive movement, social history, social justice, social work practice

In 1905, Richard C. Cabot, a physician on the staff of Massachusetts General Hospital, initiated the first medical social work program in the United States. Based on the writings of Cabot and other medical social work pioneers, this article presents the ideas that informed the early history of medical social work in the United States. In particular, this article will explore the goals and functions of early medical social work, the domestic and international contexts in which it developed, and the relationship of medical social work to the progressive movement of which it was a part. Cabot and the early medical social workers were quite explicit about their motives and goals. Unlike some recent histories of social work, which provide critical analyses of the underlying meaning of social work action (Margolin, 1997), the statements of Cabot and the other writers discussed in this article will be taken at their face value. The chapter is part of a larger project to explore the origins of social work practice in a variety of settings as conceptualized by early practitioners (see, for example, Stuart, 1986, and Stuart, 1997).

In 1905, social work, long viewed as a volunteer activity, was becoming a paid occupation (Lubove, 1965). Only a handful of professional schools existed and the first attempts to standardize the content of professional education would not be made for several decades. Abraham Flexner's (1915) famous declaration that social work was not a profession was still a decade away. A physician, not a member of the new occupation, initiated medical social work. Richard Cabot was related to members of Massachusetts General's Board of Trustees and held a faculty position at the Harvard School of Medicine. He was internationally famous as the author of the first book on hematology written in English. Appointed Physician to Outpatients at Massachusetts General in 1898, he was overwhelmed by the large number of outpatients who presented complex and difficult medical and social problems. A former director of the Boston Children's Aid Society and a consulting physician at the Massachusetts State Industrial School for Girls, Cabot knew the approaches and methods used by the emerging profession of social work (Lubove, 1965).

Hospitals in 1905 were conservative institutions, as they are today. For its first fourteen years, the social service department at Massachusetts General Hospital was not well accepted by the medical or nursing staffs. Medical social workers were confined to working with outpatients only. In addition, the social service department had few paid staff members and was privately supported by Cabot and other contributors. The department relied on volunteers and students from the Boston School for Social Workers, which had been founded in 1904 (Shoemaker, 1998), to supplement the efforts of a small paid staff. Not until 1919 were social workers made a part of the Massachusetts General Hospital staff, in spite of their sponsorship by a prominent and well-connected physician.

The Massachusetts General social work program was one of a number of similar social work programs developed in hospitals during the first decade of the twentieth century. In 1907, for example, Johns Hopkins Hospital initiated a social services department (Brogden, 1964). In the same year, the Free Synagogue, a Reform "synagogue of life and light" in New York City founded by Rabbi Stephen Wise, established a Social Service Department, directed by Sidney E. Goldstein, a rabbi and a social worker. The Social Service Department was housed in Bellevue Hospital, the major public hospital serving New York City. It provided medical social services to hospital inpatients and outpatients from the Lower East Side (Platt, 2002). By 1910, thirty hospitals in the United States had organized social service departments (Pelton, 1910). Because of its prominence and the vigor of its leadership, the Massachusetts General social service program was known as the "Rock of Gibraltar" for medical social work in the United States (Cannon, 1946, p. 48).

GOALS OF EARLY MEDICAL SOCIAL WORK

Cabot's goals for the social work program at Massachusetts General Hospital included the promotion of public health, the provision of care for large masses of patients, and the humanization of the increasingly impersonal and cold hospital environment (Cabot, 1911). Public health measures were especially important to Cabot, who particularly wanted to introduce prevention into the everyday work of the hospital. "Every case of disease," Cabot wrote, "is . . . an opportunity for the prevention of further disease through the opportunities which it affords for instruction to the sufferer and to his family and friends. . . . The social worker . . . [does] the work of hygienic instruction for . . . the preventable diseases. . . . Such teaching . . . is usually more effective in the home" (p. 469). Unlike physicians, who were busy and overworked, social workers could go outside of the hospital or clinic, into the patient's environment, to gather information or to directly intervene with the patient or in his or her environment. (See Taft, 1918, for a parallel function of the social worker in a psychiatric service.)

Social workers could also deal with problems of industrial hygiene, a field that was emerging in large part because of the contributions of social workers (Addams, 1930). "The social worker is not content with following up the radiating suggestions of possible disease in other members of the family of each patient," Cabot (1911) wrote: "The other members of the trade, perhaps similarly exposed to disease, loom up before her vision. . . . If [industrial conditions are potentially harmful], it is the business of the social worker to advertise these facts and to do what she can to change them" (p. 469).

This emphasis on public health fit well with emerging views in American medicine during "the golden age of public health" (Trattner, 1999, p. 145). "Physicians are, just now, undergoing a process of conversion or regeneration whereby the interest of the general public is becoming paramount in their work," Cabot (1911) wrote: "They come in time to look on each patient, not only as an opportunity for diagnosis and treatment, not only as a subject for medical instruction, but still more as a symptom of some disease in the community which, from the social point of view, is far more important than the individual sufferer" (p. 469).

Another motive involved the humanization of the hospital environment. Cabot (1911) believed that social workers were "needed in the hospital to make the place less grim, to keep the standard of good manners and decency higher than it otherwise tends to be, to bring to bear upon hospital routine and hospital management the criticism of a friendly, yet keen-sighted, observer, and to focus upon each individual patient all the forces of helpfulness existing in the charities, the churches, the labor unions, lodges, and other voluntary associations, as well as the opportunities for recreation and education of which the patient may be especially in need" (p. 467).

This emphasis on creating a more humane atmosphere fit well with progressive era social work interests. Like other social work specializations housed in non-social work organizations, the mission of social workers was to individualize the client while socializing the host institution (Stuart, 1986). Ida Cannon, who joined the social service department in 1906 as a student in the Boston School for Social Work and became headworker in 1907, was a nurse who became interested in social work after hearing Jane Addams speak (Bartlett, 1975). Citing Addams' 1907 address to the American Hospital Association, Cannon articulated the goal of medical social work in the following words: "The patient who is the recipient of the skilled care of doctors and nurses should be understood in his personal needs as well." She went on to emphasize "the major importance of 'trivial things'" (Cannon, 1938, p. 74).

Another early medical social worker, Sidney E. Goldstein (1910), Director of Social Service at New York's Free Synagogue, described the goals of medical social work in similar terms. Hospital social service "is destined to aid somewhat, first of all, in the resocialization of the hospital. All our so-called social institutions are being resocialized–the school, the church, the reformatory, the insurance company, the government. All these institutions that were originally called into being to meet some special social need and that have now drifted aloof, are being forced into renewed contact with society." Hospital social service would assist in "re-statement of sickness as a social problem . . . With [social] histories in our hands we shall be able to study sickness and its causes, and we shall also learn something of its social consequences. A new territory will then be opened to us for exploration" (pp. 347-348).

The resocialization of public institutions was a part of the larger progressive movement that emphasized making large institutions more responsive to the society. Responding to demographic and social changes, American progressives believed that increasing the responsiveness of institutions to people would further the twin goals of social justice and efficiency (Kirschner, 1975). Thus, medical social work was a response to social changes affecting all American institutions in the early twentieth century.

THE CONTEXT OF EARLY MEDICAL SOCIAL WORK

In 1905, Massachusetts General Hospital was in the midst of a transition from a charity institution, serving the poor, to a modern medical institution, devoted to the treatment of the sick from all social classes (Vogel, 1980). The famous Flexner report on medical education (1910) exemplified this change.

The report, which exerted tremendous influence on the development of medical education in the United States, called for a medical curriculum based on scientific investigation, controlled observation of the patient in the hospital environment, and clinical training for medical students.

In part, the transition to the modern hospital resulted from the revolution in medical knowledge that occurred during the nineteenth century. Hospitals became safer places as the result of the development of antiseptic techniques. New diagnostic tools, such as the x-ray and the stethoscope, improved the ability of hospital-based physicians to diagnose and treat diseases. New scientific discoveries made new treatments possible that promised to expedite the cure of disease. While some contemporaries criticized these developments as dehumanizing, the improved ability of the hospital-based physician to observe and isolate the causes of disease enabled modern hospitals to provide, in Cabot's words, "Better Doctoring for Less Money" (Cabot, 1917).

As a result of these changes the number of hospitals increased rapidly in the early twentieth century. "Few municipalities of any size now exist without their city hospitals," wrote Herbert R. Howard, the superintendent of Massachusetts General Hospital and chairman of the newly formed American Medical Association's Section on Hospitals in 1913. The modern hospital should stand for three things, according to Howard:

1. the care of the patients,
2. scientific investigation, and
3. the education of physicians, nurses, orderlies, every one within its walls, and through them the community at large, concerning the various maladies that are brought within its doors (p. 1965).

To do this, not only a physical examination and prescription of treatment was necessary, but also "an investigation of [the patient's] ability to apply the treatment," usually involving a home visit (Howard, 1913, p. 1965). Thus, in less than a decade, a leading hospital administrator had accepted the role of social work in a hospital setting.

The ability of the hospital to communicate with patients and help them apply the prescribed treatments was complicated by widespread social and demographic change. Immigration had an enormous effect upon the educational and health institutions of American cities in the late nineteenth and early twentieth centuries. Between 1905 and 1914 as many as a million persons per year were arriving in the United States from Europe annually, many of them settling in Eastern and Midwestern cities. Immigration was accompanied in the United States by large-scale internal migration from rural areas to cities. By the first decade of the twentieth century, Eastern and Southern Europe had replaced Northwestern Europe as major sources of immigrants (Bureau of the Census, 1975, Series C 89-119). Language and cultural differences complicated the adjustment of these new immigrants to American society even as changes in the economy threatened members of the older American elite. Population growth and urban crowding in was unprecedented in the experience of most Americans.

Between 1890 and 1920, Boston's population grew from 484,780 to 748,060. Although the proportion of foreign-born persons in the population declined somewhat, from 34.7% to 31.9%, the composition of the immigrant population changed. Before 1880, most immigrants who settled in Boston had come from Ireland and Canada (Handlin, 1969). Between 1890 and 1910, increasing numbers of immigrants arrived from Eastern and Southern Europe. By 1920, although Ireland and Canada still contributed the largest percentage of the foreign-born white population (23.8 and 17.6 per cent, respectively), Russia and Italy each contributed 15.9 per cent (Bureau of the Census, 1922, pp. 50-52).

The arrival of members of "the newer Catholic races"–French, Germans, Italians, Syrians, Lithuanian, Poles, and Portuguese–strained the largely Irish Roman Catholic Boston establishment (O'Toole, 1992, pp. 120-121). Other immigrants, including many from Eastern Europe, were Jewish. For the Boston Protestant establishment, the arrival of immigrants from Eastern and Southern Europe was similarly difficult. As historian James O'Toole (1992) commented,

> Ever since the middle of the [nineteenth] century, immigration and ethnicity had never been very far beneath the surface of everyday life in Boston and its environs. The region, which had had a remarkably homogeneous population throughout the colonial era, was now expected to assimilate vast numbers of foreigners, most of whom were markedly different in their ethnic backgrounds and religious practices. Little wonder that the native population resorted to the language of natural disaster, speaking of immigrant "floods" and "tidal waves," to describe the changes. (p. 118)

In such a situation the danger of negative stereotyping was great, particularly in organizations serving immigrant populations that were staffed and directed by native born people–schools, the justice system, hospitals, and factories. "We are dealing with people in masses so great that the individual is lost sight of," Cabot (1919) wrote. "The individual becomes reduced to a type, a case, a specimen of a class." There was a "danger of dehumanization." The individualization of the person in such situations was a critical task of the social worker and a key reason for the profession's growth. "Above all of her duties it is the function of the social worker to discover and to provide for those individual needs which are otherwise in danger of being lost sight of" (p. viii).

INTERNATIONAL INFLUENCES

As Daniel T. Rodgers (1998) reminds us, social reform was an international matter a century ago. International conferences, like the contemporary International Conference on Social Work in Health and Mental Health, were held on a variety of topics, and observers on both sides of the Atlantic followed changes in the organization of hospitals as well as many other topics. Cabot and the other American pioneers of medical social work were inspired by developments in European health care that emphasized the community context of disease.

Cabot was aware of the London Charity Organisation Society's (COS) experiment in medical social work. In 1895, the London COS placed one of its district secretaries in the Royal Free Hospital to investigate the ability to pay of patients presenting themselves for treatment and to link the hospital with other charities in the community (Lubove, 1965). The initial interest of the English "Lady Almoners" in financial investigation of the patient soon gave way to an interest in the patient's adjustment to disease (Cabot, 1919). American medical social workers recognized the "Lady Almoners" as the forerunners of their specialization ("English Almoner Visiting United States and Canada," 1946; Read, 1946).

Other European experiments in health care service delivery were relevant as well. In his discussion of the precursors of the Massachusetts General Hospital social work program, Cabot (1919) mentioned the work of Dr. Calmette of Lille, who used home visitors to link his dispensary and the home of the patient. "The home visitor was a part of the plan of anti-sepsis, a method of destroying the bacteria through disinfection and sterilization of the premises and of the patient's linen. In America the work of the home visitor . . . has been concerned less with the disinfection and bactericidal procedures than with the positive measures of hygiene, such as the better housing of the patient, better nutrition, better provision for sunlight and fresh air, and above all instruction of the patient as to the nature of his disease and the methods to be pursued in combating it" (p. xv). Another French experiment separated children from the neighborhood of tuberculous parents or other tuberculous persons. Children were especially susceptible to tuberculous infection, so this approach indicated an "active or aggressive attitude" toward the patient's environment on the part of the physician, the possibility of "truly preventive action" (pp. xviii-xix).

Cabot and Cannon were actively involved in international consultation and made presentations to international forums. Cabot's classic, *Social Work: Essays on the Meeting-Ground of Doctor and Social Work* (1919) was originally presented as a series of lectures at the Sorbonne. Cabot gave a series of lectures on medical social work in Paris in 1927 and participated in the First International Conference of Social Work held in Paris in 1928. Cannon presented a paper at the Second International Conference at Frankfurt in 1932 (Cannon, 1946).

SOCIAL JUSTICE AND EFFICIENCY

The Progressive era preoccupation with social justice and efficiency found an echo in Cabot's goal to humanize the hospital as an institution and prevent disease. In many host institutions, social work's mission was to socialize the institution and individualize the client (Stuart, 1986). Medical social workers explained the social world of the patient to the physician. They also promoted public health measures in the community, improving the patient's environment to eliminate the causes of disease. Garnet Pelton (1910), the first director of the social service program at Massachusetts General Hospital, wrote that "prevention rather than cure is the watchword" of the modern hospital, "hygiene rather than drugs" (p. 333).

An important motive for medical social work, according to Cabot (1919) was the increasing use of scientific method, resulting in more accurate and precise diagnoses, time consuming examinations, specialization, search for underlying causes of symptoms, including "radical and detailed knowledge of [the] patient's life outside the dispensary" followed by increasingly complex treatments. The increasing complexity of medical practice and the consequent dehumanization of the patient pervaded the hospital and provided a powerful motive for developing the medical social work specialization.

Prevention provided a second motive. Preventive medicine had the potential to isolate and conquer a disease and made hospitals important resources for persons from all social classes, not only for the poor. "From the institution of tuberculosis dispensaries with their home visitors in America," Cabot (1919) wrote, "the poverty of the individual ceased to be a necessary badge for admission. Especially since many of our dispensaries have been instituted and maintained by the State, and therefore are paid for by all its citizens in their taxes, any one so unfortunate as to acquire tuberculosis, or be suspected of it, feels himself wholly justified in seeking help at a State-maintained tuberculosis dispensary" (p. xvii). The result was "the disregarding of property lines" (p. xviii), the abandonment of the means test as a prerequisite for service. Like other social workers in specialized settings, the focus of the medical social worker was on the setting's social task, in this case the promotion of health, not on the client's poverty (Stuart, 1999).

The Functions of the Medical Social Worker

As in other social work specializations, social diagnosis became the central activity of the medical social worker. Pelton (1910) wrote that "the aim of hospital social work is the social diagnosis, prognosis and treatment of the hospital's or dispensary's sick poor wherever the need is indicated" (p. 332). Cabot (1919) developed an outline for the social diagnosis that included the individual and his or her environment (see Table 1). He commented:

> To make a social diagnosis we should make a summary statement about the individual in his environment. That summary is to include his mental and physical state, and the physical and mental characteristics of his environment. (I here use the word "mental" to include everything that is not physical; that is, to include the moral, the spiritual, every influence that does not come under physics or chemistry.) (p. 109)

A leading medical ethicist, Cabot was suspicious of institutional solutions to human problems (O'Brien, 1985). Rather than a proponent of an increasingly reductionist medicine, as he is sometimes portrayed (Vogel, 1980), Cabot was fundamentally an individualist. Cabot believed that individualization, rather than programmatic solutions would solve the problems of an increasingly impersonal world. In this respect, as in many others, Cabot's beliefs were consonant with the American progressive movement's suspicion of big government.

In spite of their emphasis on environmental intervention, many of early medical social work leaders had an anti-institutional bias; they were suspicious of large-scale solutions for what they saw as fundamentally individual problems. Consequently, methods for promoting individual adaptation developed more rapidly than methods for inducing environmental change. Since they served patients because of their diseases rather than their poverty, medical social workers were among the first to provide social work services to the non-poor. A focus on the individual in social work practice, promoted during the 1920s by psychiatric social workers, was endorsed by

TABLE 1. Guide for Social Diagnosis at Massachusetts General Hospital (1919)

Diagnosis Shall Characterize:

I. The Individual
  1. Physical
    a. Heredity.
    b. Health.
  2. Mental
    a. Mental deficiency.
    b. Mental disease.
    c. Temperament. Character.

II. His Environment
  1. Physical
    a. Food. Clothes. Housing.
    b. Industrial conditions.
    c. School conditions.
    d. Climate. Natural beauty or ugliness.
  2. Mental
    a. Family and friends.
    b. Education. Play.
    c. Religion.

Source: Richard C. Cabot, *Social Work: Essays on the Meeting-Ground of Doctor and Social Worker*. Boston: Houghton Mifflin, 1919, p. 109.

many medical social workers (Stuart, 1997). Indeed, Cabot himself endorsed the interest in psychiatric social work that followed World War I. "This psychiatric eruption," he said in 1919, "is the best thing that has happened in social work during the last thirty years" (quoted in Woodroofe, 1971, p. 128).

CONCLUSION

This chapter described the ideas of Richard Cabot and other early leaders of medical social work. Despite their anti-institutional focus, they emphasized the importance for medical institutions to take into account both the individual and his or her environment. Medical social work was part of the progressive movement of the early twentieth century in the United States; at the same time, it was part of an international social reform movement.

Today, as a century ago, we are experiencing another era of international-ization. The causes of the two episodes of globalization are similar. Com-merce is increasingly international, as it was in the late nineteenth and early twentieth century. Today, as a century ago, globalization is the result of im-provements in transportation and communication. As at the turn of the last century, international exchange is increasing, spurred by the similar develop-ments occurring around the world as a result of similar stimuli (Drucker, 1999). The International Conference on Social Work in Health and Mental Health has met three times since its inaugural meeting in Jerusalem in 1995. The number of other international social work conferences increased during the 1990s as professionals sought to understand similar worldwide develop-ments.

One cannot help being struck by the rollback of welfare state benefits, not only in the United States but also in many other former welfare states. Nations that never were able to provide extensive benefits to their citizens are today encouraged to explore market-based solutions to social problems. In the United States and elsewhere, new views of welfare and the role of government are emerging. Managed care, cost containment, and privatization are the watchwords of social policy in this post-welfare state era (Gilbert, 1995; Midgley, 1999).

The dual focus of the early medical social workers on the person and on his or her environment, on the patient and on public health, is needed today, per-haps more than ever. Ironically, the medicalization of social problems in con-temporary times has resulted in a focus on individual pathology rather than social causation in health, even as the rising cost and complexity of health care systems challenge consumers. As was the case a century ago, lifestyle issues are implicated as impacting the health status of persons worldwide. The im-portance of understanding the patient's cultural milieu is underscored today by recognition of the importance of spirituality to the healing process. Reaf-firming the environmental emphasis of medical social work pioneers provides a way for today's health care social workers to incorporate environmental modification into their practice and promote the health of all citizens.

REFERENCES

Addams, J. (1930). Social workers and the other professions. *Proceedings of the Na-tional Conference of Social Work, 57*, 50-54.

Bartlett, H. M. (1975). Ida M. Cannon: Pioneer in medical social work. *Social Service Review, 49*, 2, 208-229.

Brogden, M. S. (1964). The Johns Hopkins Hospital Department of Social Service, 1907-31. *Social Service Review, 38*, 1, 88-98.

Bureau of the Census (1922). *Population, 1920. 14th Census of the United States, Volume III: Composition and Characteristics of the Population by States.* Washington, D. C.: Government Printing Office.

Bureau of the Census (1975). *Historical Statistics of the United States: Colonial Times to 1970, Bicentennial Edition, Part 1.* Washington, D. C.: Government Printing Office.

Cabot, R. C. (1911). Social service work in hospitals. *Annals of the American Academy of Political and Social Science, 37,* 2, 467-471.

Cabot, R. C. (1915). *Social Service and the Art of Healing.* New York: Moffat, Yard, and Company.

Cabot, R. C. (1916). Better doctoring for less money. *American Magazine, 81* (April): 7-9, 77-81; *81* (May): 43-44, 76-81.

Cabot, R. C. (1919). *Social Work: Essays on the Meeting-Ground of Doctor and Social Worker.* Boston: Houghton Mifflin.

Cannon, I. M. (1938). Twenty years of our association–Its significance to our professional growth. *Bulletin of the American Association of Medical Social Workers, 11,* 6, 73-82.

Cannon, M. A. (1946). Ida Cannon and medical social work. *Bulletin of the American Association of Medical Social Workers 19,* 3, 47-50.

Drucker, P. (1999). Beyond the information revolution. *Atlantic Monthly, 284,* 4 (October), 47-57.

"English Almoner Visiting United States and Canada" (1946). *Bulletin of the American Association of Medical Social Workers, 19,* 2, 38.

Flexner, A. (1910). *Medical Education in the United States and Canada: A Report to the Carnegie Foundation for the Advancement of Teaching.* New York: Arno Press, 1972.

Flexner, A. (1915). Is social work a profession? *Proceedings of the National Conference of Charities and Corrections, 42,* 576-590.

Gilbert, N. (1995). *Welfare Justice: Restoring Social Equity.* New Haven: Yale University Press.

Goldstein, S. E. (1910). Hospital Social Service; Principles and Implications. *Proceedings, National Conference of Charities and Correction,* 341-348.

Handlin, O. (1969). *Boston's Immigrants: A Study in Acculturation.* New York: Atheneum.

Howard, H. B. (1910). Growth and efficiency of hospitals. *Journal of the American Medical Association, 61,* 22 (November 29): 1965-1966.

Kirschner, D. S. (1975). The ambiguous legacy: Social justice and social control in the Progressive Era. *Historical Reflections, 2,* 1, 69-88.

Lubove, R. (1965). *The Professional Altruist: The Emergence of Social Work as a Career, 1880-1930.* Cambridge, Massachusetts: Harvard University Press.

Margolin, L. (1997). *Under the Cover of Kindness: The Invention of Social Work.* Charlottesville: University Press of Virginia.

Midgley, J. (1999). Growth, redistribution, and welfare: Toward social investment. *Social Service Review, 73,* 1, 3-21.

O'Brien, L. (1985). "A bold plunge into the sea of values": The career of Dr. Richard Cabot. *New England Quarterly, 58,* 4, 533-553.

O'Toole, J. M. (1992). "The newer Catholic races": Ethnic Catholicism in Boston, 1900-1940. *New England Quarterly, 65,* 1, 117-134.

Pelton, G. I. (1910). The History and Status of Hospital Social Work. *Proceedings, National Conference of Charities and Correction,* 332-341.

Platt, C. (2002). *Stephen Wise Free Synagogue: The First Ninety Years.* Retrieved September 25, 2002, from *http://www.swfs.org/History.htm.*

Read, B. (1946). Medical social work as seen by a British almoner. *Bulletin of the American Association of Medical Social Workers, 20,* 6, 69-74.

Rodgers, D. T. (1998). *Atlantic Crossings: Social Politics in a Progressive Age.* Cambridge, Massachusetts: Harvard University Press.

Rosen, G. (1976). The efficiency criterion in medical care, 1900-1920. *Bulletin of the History of Medicine, 50,* 1, 28-44.

Shoemaker, L. M. (1998). Early conflicts in social work education. *Social Service Review 72,* 182-191.

Stuart, P. (1986). School social work as a professional segment: Continuity in transitional times. *Social Work in Education 8,* 3, 141-153.

Stuart, P. H. (1997). Community care and the origins of psychiatric social work. *Social Work in Health Care, 25,* 3, 35-36.

Stuart, P. H. (1999). "In a world gone industrial": Specialization and the search for social work practice above the poverty line. In *The Professionalization of Poverty: Social Work and the Poor in the Twentieth Century,* edited by G. R. Lowe and P. N. Reid. (Pp. 51-61.) New York: Aldine de Gruyter.

Taft, J. (1918). The limitations of the psychiatrist. *Medicine and Surgery, 2,* 365-367.

Trattner, W. I. (1999). *From Poor Law to Welfare State: A History of Social Welfare in America,* 6th edition. New York: Free Press.

Vogel, M. J. (1980). *The Invention of the Modern Hospital: Boston, 1870-1930.* Chicago: University of Chicago Press.

Woodroofe, K. (1971). *From Charity to Social Work in England and the United States.* Toronto: University of Toronto Press.

Doing It Well:
An Empirical Study of Expertise
in Mental Health Social Work

Martin Ryan
Bill Healy
Noel Renouf

SUMMARY. Social workers are being challenged internationally to be accountable by defining competency standards at beginning and advanced levels. The study that is the subject of this article will develop the work of one of the authors, which involved a 5-year longitudinal study of beginning social workers and another of experienced social workers. These studies resulted in a book on professional expertise (Fook, Ryan, &

Martin Ryan, PhD, (martin.ryan@latrobe.edu.au) is Senior Lecturer, School of Social Work & Social Policy, La Trobe University, Melbourne, Victoria 3086 Australia. Bill Healy, MA, (b.healy@latrobe.edu.au) is Associate Professor in Mental Health and Social Work, School of Social Work & Social Policy, La Trobe University, Melbourne, Victoria 3086 Australia & North Western Mental Health. Noel Renouf, PhD, (n.renouf@latrobe.edu.au) is Senior Social Work Advisor, North Western Mental Health, and Adjunct Senior Lecturer, La Trobe University, Melbourne, Victoria 3086 Australia.

The authors would like to thank the social workers in the North-West Mental Health Program for their generous cooperation and participation in the study, and Professor Allan Borowski for the financial assistance made available by the School of Social Work & Social Policy at La Trobe University.

[Haworth co-indexing entry note]: "Doing It Well: An Empirical Study of Expertise in Mental Health Social Work." Ryan, Martin, Bill Healy, and Noel Renouf. Co-published simultaneously in *Social Work in Mental Health* (The Haworth Social Work Practice Press, an imprint of The Haworth Press, Inc.) Vol. 2, No. 2/3, 2004, pp. 21-37; and: *Social Work Approaches in Health and Mental Health from Around the Globe* (ed: Metteri et al.) The Haworth Social Work Practice Press, an imprint of The Haworth Press, Inc., 2004, pp. 21-37. Single or multiple copies of this article are available for a fee from The Haworth Document Delivery Service [1-800-HAWORTH, 9:00 a.m. - 5:00 p.m. (EST). E-mail address: docdelivery@haworthpress.com].

Digital Object Identifier: 10.1300/J200v2n02_03

Hawkins, 2000). The present study furthered that work and subjected this theory of professional expertise to further testing by examining the work of a sample of expert (rather than experienced) social workers in the mental health field in Melbourne, Australia. Data was collected from a selected sample of mental health social workers by the use of focus group interview. This article reports on the study's findings and discusses their significance and application. *[Article copies available for a fee from The Haworth Document Delivery Service: 1-800-HAWORTH. E-mail address: <docdelivery@haworthpress.com> Website: <http://www.HaworthPress.com> © 2004 by The Haworth Press, Inc. All rights reserved.]*

KEYWORDS. Expertise, expert social work, mental health social work practice

INTRODUCTION

Given the changing international climate of welfare service provision which is increasingly characterised by the breakdown of the welfare state, the spread of economic rationalism and globalisation, and a growing trend towards deprofessionalisation, there is a need to identify and examine exactly what social work professionals can do and what they are skilled at. This has implications both nationally and internationally for professional social work education, the provision of health and welfare services, and the profession's place in those services.

Although some research on competency has been conducted (Vass, 1996; O'Hagen, 1996; Campbell, 1996), there is a strong need to link competency research findings with a number of questions of broader concern to the social work profession, particularly those working in health and mental health, and professional education such as: What constitutes professional expertise? How do you develop and educate for it? What is the nature of the relationship to theory and practice? What is the nature of both generic and specialist social work expertise? What is the nature of social work expertise in the health and mental health fields?

This paper reports on a research study that sought to answer the key question of: What constitutes expertise in mental health social work? The study examined the practice of a sample of ten expert social workers in the mental health field in Melbourne, Australia. The study utilised small group interviews in which the social workers described and discussed "memorable practice situations."

LITERATURE REVIEW

The study of expertise and 'expert' practice is a controversial endeavour. Professions have been criticised for their dominance and disempowerment of the clients they are ostensibly serving (Leonard, 1998). Professions therefore have a vested interest in identifying and controlling the definition of expertise (Larson, 1990).

In addition to this political dimension, there is the problem of there being no agreed upon definition of 'expert' and 'expertise' (Benbenishty, 1992). Some studies have attempted to do this, most particularly studies of 'expert' systems in computer science (Wakefield, 1990), which attempted to map the cognitive skills of 'experts' for the development of computer systems. These studies have been criticised for their inability to map features of human reasoning that cannot be articulated easily, and that are, in turn, important parts of human decision-making in complex situations (Dreyfus & Dreyfus, 1986).

Dreyfus and Dreyfus (1986) have developed a model of skill acquisition that provides a framework for mapping changes in thinking as a professional learns how to act in unstructured situations. This model has achieved wide acknowledgment in a number of disciplines (Eraut, 1994). They identified five stages (novice, advanced beginner, competent, proficient, expert) through which the learner advances.

The Dreyfus and Dreyfus model served as the framework for the work of Fook, Ryan, and Hawkins on professional expertise based on a series of studies from 1990 onwards (Fook, Ryan, & Hawkins, 1994; Ryan, Fook, & Hawkins, 1995; Fook, Ryan & Hawkins, 1997a; Fook, Ryan, & Hawkins, 1997b; Hawkins, Fook, & Ryan, 2001). The entire series of studies resulted in a book (Fook, Ryan, & Hawkins, 2000) in which a theory about how expertise is learnt and developed was postulated. This theory was specifically developed for practice which dealt with complexities and uncertainties in making and taking value- and knowledge-based decisions and actions in changing situations, and some specific features involved in this expertise were described. Both the substantive and procedural knowledge necessary in these competencies was described, and these descriptions were inductively formulated from practitioners' own conceptualisations of concrete practices.

The empirical studies in Fook et al. (2000) primarily consisted of: (1) a 5-year longitudinal study of 40 beginning social work students through their two years of social work education (Bachelor of Social Work degree) and their first three years of practice; and (2) an accompanying study of 30 experienced social workers. These studies were all qualitative in design, and relied on the use of responses to practice vignettes, and a description of critical incidents from the respondents' own practice collected in individual interviews.

Fook et al. (2000) were able to develop the five stage Dreyfus and Dreyfus model by adding two further stages to the model, that of pre-student and experienced. They were also to identify dimensions of expertise development. These were:

1. Knowledge (substantive)–types of facts or systems of ideas which were evident in practice;
2. Knowledge (procedural)–types of knowledge used and devised to make substantive knowledge applicable;
3. Skills–"what they are confident in doing" (Fook et al., 2000, p. 18)
4. Values–"ideals and beliefs as to how the world should be and how people should normally act" (Fook et al., 2000, p. 18)
5. Contextuality–extent to which practitioners were context bound (domain specific) and the degree to which they were aware of contexts and how they were conceptualised;
6. Reflexivity–degree to which practitioners were able to locate themselves in their contexts as responsible agents and the degree to which they felt empowered to act;
7. Breadth of vision–refers to the degree to which practitioners identified with a vision of service which extended beyond the parameters of an employed position;
8. Flexibility ("ability to generate a range of options, including those which are not possible in that particular context" (Fook et al., 2000, p. 188) and creativity (to be ". . . to devise new categories of understanding and strategies appropriate to them" (Fook et al., 2000, p. 188)
9. Use of theory (formal)
10. Approach–refers to the initial lens through which practitioners view situations, whether through the viewpoint of the individual, or from a broader perspective.
11. Perspective on profession–orientation to the profession and development of a professional identity.

THE PRESENT STUDY

Aims

The broad aims of the present study were first, to further build upon the general theory of expertise expounded by Fook et al. (2000) and second, to extend it by investigating its applicability in a particular social work setting.

Therefore, the present study sought to advance the previous work undertaken by Fook et al. (2000) by:

1. conducting further empirical work to subject the theory of professional expertise to further testing and refinement by examining the work of expert social work practitioners in a specific field, viz. mental health;
2. focussing on expert rather than just experienced practitioners as previous studies had done;
3. utilising small group interviews rather than just individual interviews again as previous studies had done.

Thus the specific aims of the study were:

1. to subject the theory of professional expertise to further testing by examining the work of expert social workers in a specific field;
2. to further investigate the applicability of the theory by the use of group interviews.

The previous studies collected data through interviews with individuals. There was a need for further research utilising different methods to access the practice of expert social workers. In order to do this, small group interviews designed to facilitate interaction and dialogue amongst respondents were undertaken.

The major significance of the present study lies in the fact that it seeks to further develop an existing theory of professional expertise through continuing empirical testing. This was intended to strengthen the robustness of the theory that has direct applicability in professional education, in promoting the role of the profession and curriculum design, especially at Masters and professional doctorate levels.

METHODOLOGY

The study examined the practice of a sample of expert social workers in the mental health field in Melbourne, Australia. 'Expert' social workers were defined as those whose practice is considered expert by their peers and supervisors and who have had more than 5 years of practice. This judgement was ascertained by asking all social workers within an area-based mental health program to nominate (via a simple questionnaire) peers and supervisors to whom they would go for advice in solving a problem and who they would consider to be excellent supervisors.

The questionnaire was mailed out to all 67 social workers in North Western Mental Health in Melbourne, which employs social workers in comprehensive community based specialist and generalist services across the whole spectrum from acute wards to outreach services for long-term clients, from early intervention with young adults to work with aged persons. In particular, this population of social workers was chosen for several specific reasons that were believed to strengthen the capacity of the research study to realise its aims: first, there was a strong interest in the project expressed by the social workers; second, ease of access (one of the researchers is a senior social worker in this service); and third, because these social workers work in the same organisation, it can be assumed that they have knowledge of each others' level of professional capacities.

The letter accompanying the questionnaire asked the respondents to identify up to five social workers from within the Mental Health Program whom they regarded as expert practitioners. In this letter, they were offered some broad criteria to assist them with their judgments: "For example, such a person may be someone whose work you may have confidence in, someone who you would go to for supervision, someone to whom you would go for help with a practice problem or someone you would ask to help someone you know."

A total of 45 questionnaires were returned (67% response rate). After scrutinising the returns, it was decided that the ten social workers who were nominated most frequently by their peers would be invited to participate in the study. The identified expert practitioners were then interviewed in small focus groups of 2 to 4 persons, usually with two researchers present. The social workers were asked in advance to be prepared to talk with their peers about "memorable practice situations" drawn from their experiences. These focus group interviews were audiotaped and transcribed verbatim.

The analysis of the interview data was done both deductively and inductively. The deductive analysis comprised a content analysis of responses in relation to the theory of expertise developed by Fook et al. (2000). It specifically examined:

- what types of knowledge (substantive or procedural) were used by respondents, including what types of concepts, theories;
- what types of skills were used?
- what values, or value-based assumptions, were implicitly or explicitly expressed by respondents?
- what types of approaches or theoretical or political orientations were explicitly or implicitly expressed by respondents?
- what evidence is there of rule-based thinking, the ability to prioritise, detached or analytical perspectives, the use of intuition?
- how did work context appear to influence practice?

The inductive aspect of the analysis focused on the themes and issues raised by the practitioners, and built up a picture of practice as conceptualised by the professionals themselves. For this aspect of the analysis, a broad thematic analysis (Kellehear, 1993) was conducted. In places however, when a more specific issue was investigated in-depth, the analysis was semiotic (Kellehear, 1993), focusing in particular on implicit assumptions, gaps and silences in the accounts.

RESULTS

The results of the study will be presented as follows: (1) the characteristics of the study's sample; (2) brief descriptions will be provided of the respondents' "memorable practice situations"; (3) the results of the content analysis of the data will be briefly presented; and (4) an outline of the themes that emerged from the thematic analysis of the data.

SAMPLE CHARACTERISTICS

The sample of ten social workers came from the following areas from within the program: (1) four were in community mental health teams for adults with serious mental illness; (2) three were in aged persons psychiatry; (3) one was in an adult acute inpatient unit; (4) another in a crisis assessment and treatment team; and (5) the remaining person was from a specialist service for early psychosis.

In terms of qualifications and experience, the entire sample had the basic social work qualification (Bachelor of Social Work), which is the common standard credential for professional social work in Australia. In addition, two had a postgraduate, i.e., postqualifying, social work qualification (Master of Social Work) and three were undertaking postgraduate qualifications or had incomplete postgraduate qualifications. The range of years of experience since qualifying as a social worker varied from eight to 31 years, with a mean of 17 years. There was a mean of ten years work in mental health, and seven of the ten had also worked in other fields of social work.

MEMORABLE PRACTICE SITUATIONS

The social workers reported a considerable range of "memorable practice situations":

1. work with a young man experiencing first episode psychosis and his family;

2. consultation with nursing home staff about an elderly man with Huntington's Disease;
3. work with a young man with dual diagnosis who subsequently suicided;
4. work with a woman with borderline personality disorder (bpd), with a good outcome;
5. a single session with a depressed man, focused on budgeting;
6. work with an elderly woman with borderline personality disorder;
7. work with another, younger woman with borderline personality disorder, with a good outcome;
8. advocacy with a public housing authority on behalf of woman with schizophrenia;
9. a session with a severely depressed woman (also with borderline personality disorder) and its aftermath; and
10. two situations presented by one social worker–first, an elderly man who suicided, and second, work with another man with lithium toxicity.

These situations covered a broad range from: (1) basic social work tasks (budgeting and advocacy with a public housing authority); (2) secondary consultation; through to (3) difficult, stressful, and dangerous situations (severe depression, dual diagnosis, threatened suicide, borderline personality disorder, and first presentation of psychosis.)

CONTENT ANALYSIS FINDINGS

The features outlined by Fook et al. (2000) for the expert stage under each of the 11 dimensions of expertise development were searched for in the descriptions of the respondents' "memorable practice situations." The results of this content analysis are outlined in Table 1. For this article, the basis of these content analysis findings will not be detailed in any depth. It was considered to be more important to focus on the newer material emerging from the thematic analysis.

As can be seen from Table One, all dimensions were considered to be evident in the respondents' interview data, bar breadth of vision (extent to which the respondents identified with a vision of service that extended beyond the boundaries of an employed position) and approach (the way in which respondents view situations, whether from the viewpoint of the individual, or from a broader perspective). Breadth of vision was noted in the respondents' accounts in that they saw cases and their work in general as opportunities for change, but other forms of continuities or stabilities such as membership of

TABLE 1. Features of the Dimensions of the Expert Stage (Fook et al., 2000) and Their Presence in the Interview Data (as Indicated by a Tick)

Dimension	Features	Presence
1. Knowledge (substantive)	Recognise multiple viewpoints Use amalgam of knowledge for new knowledge Transcends personal identification Recognise multi-faceted aspects	√
2. Knowledge (procedural)	Rework old patterns Prioritise according to broad values Transferability	√
3. Skills	Wide variety of skills Generate range of options Responsive to change and unpredictability Recast skills as contextual	√
4. Values	Broader values	√
5. Contextuality	Creative use of knowledge Transferability of knowledge Context as client Contextual knowledge development	√
6. Reflexivity	Involvement not intervention Recognise own ability to act Sense of personal power (agency)	√
7. Breadth of vision	Commitment to creating broader values Alternative forms of continuity Change framed as challenge/opportunity Prioritise prioritising re: broader values Grounded yet transcendent	
8. Flexibility and creativity	Process-oriented Risk-taking and creative Longitudinal (not lateral) prioritising	√
9. Use of theory	Create own theory Contextual theory development Critical and self-reflective Transferability not generalisability	√
10. Approach	Social distancing and more contextual/organisational orientation (experienced)	√
11. Perspective on profession	Transcendence of professional codes/rules Professionalism not defined by the job Profession as 'calling'	√

community groups or movements were not noted. In terms of approach, which had been outlined only to an experienced level by Fook et al. (2000), these respondents were clearly performing at the experienced level in that the clients they saw were viewed as individuals and in broader terms of their context and the impact on their organisation.

THEMATIC ANALYSIS FINDINGS

Analysis of the interview material revealed six additional themes that appear to be relevant to the dimensions of expertise among this group of social workers. At least among this sample, they are themes that express the approach by expert social workers to some of the particular challenges of work in the mental health field.

'The Knowledge'

Work in this field requires a great deal of specialist knowledge about mental health problems and how they are dealt with. Social workers described the application of very specific knowledge about the experiences of people with mental health problems, diagnosis, medication, treatment side effects, as well as detailed knowledge about the intricacies of a complex service system.

This is well illustrated by the following quote from a respondent:

> The fact is that there are a whole of different things at play there. There are things around his physical illness, there are things around his mental state, there are things around where he lives, there are things around the staff and how they relate to him and how they are responding to him, things about what a mental health team can do.

'A Lot of Hard Grind'

Many of the cases the experts described involved intense work in situations that are highly charged emotionally, often with significant threat of suicide and self-harm, highly 'demanding' behaviour from clients, and working with clients who are very disturbed, sometimes involving real danger to the social worker and others. There was a clear emphasis on the importance of assessing and dealing with significant risk, literally in life and death situations e.g.,

> *this is the reality of working in mental health, people do kill themselves.*

But this level of demand comes at a cost. One respondent captured the feeling of being worn down by the seemingly never ending pressure:

I do get very frustrated at times. You know 16 years or so on, I mean you get all the variety, but there are themes of course and there are patterns and some if it has gotten a bit wearing. I can't say I have the same level of enthusiasm that I used to have. And that's a bit sad because I look at some of my younger social workers and I see that and I think yeah I used to feel that way and that's really lovely. So it's not boring exactly but a certain kind of wearing down.

With many clients, progress has been slow and setbacks frequent, and the social worker has needed to combat feelings of hopelessness in the client and within the service system. These social workers were aware that there are inherent demands on their own emotional resources, and aware of the difficulty of managing their own personal and emotional experiences and responses in order to practice effectively.

This is well illustrated by the following quote from a respondent:

A lot of this stuff is very confronting and not to put too fine a point on it, provokes pretty powerful feelings in yourself.

'We Are Here for the Clients'

We are here for the clients, we work for them. I often tell the [clients] and their families they should be really critical of what I do. (Comment from a respondent)

Coupled with this knowledge is a real passion for the mental health field, as exemplified by this quote from a respondent:

(Friends) . . . get freaked out by it (mental health work) I guess, but I guess it's something you have a passion for or you don't.

The social workers spoke about their work with enthusiasm and passion for mental health issues, and, more particularly, demonstrated close involvement and investment in their clients' well being. They demonstrated the capacity to care as well as act, and to combine dedication with skill and a commitment to empowering practice with their clients. To give an example, when they spoke (as they frequently did) about involving and representing the ideas and needs of family members, they demonstrated a simultaneous concern with moral or ethical responsibility (what is just), theoretical justification (a focus on systems and knowledge of the principles of good effective practice), and technical expertise (the skills necessary to develop and maintain an effective partnership with families).

'The Complicated and the Difficult'

The expert social workers described intensely complicated and difficult practice situations, typically requiring the simultaneous consideration of different aspects of the client's situation: their mental health problems, social relationships, legal issues and issues of rights, in the context of challenging ethical and personal issues for the workers. The work required that these aspects be considered together, in their interaction, and balanced out. In some cases, the social workers were juggling multiple roles: case management, primary therapy, and secondary consultation. Significantly, this complexity was valued. "The challenge is to work out what the heck is going on here," as one said. The social workers often took a very long-term perspective while dealing with here-and-now issues. They often worked therapeutically (sometimes drawing on sophisticated therapeutic methods) while simultaneously 'getting their hands dirty' with everyday issues (such as telephoning the Office of Housing, or working with a client on their household budget).

This level of difficulty was exemplified in one instance in which a respondent called a situation "moderately difficult" when it involved:

> *making judgment[s] . . . about risk issues, safety issues, symptom issues, the least restrictive environment this person should be in.*

In order to do this work, the social workers have had to overcome the fear of both physical and psychological threat, and have to be able to 'work on the edge,' accepting responsibility for the risk, often for long periods of time.

> *It's almost a mantra when you're in a team–document, document, document. Do the risk assessment–document, document, document. You need to be able protect yourself if you go into the Coroner's Court.*

> probably most of . . . the clients that I . . . see because they are such high risk . . . I am doing risk assessment . . . At what point do you say: OK, it does need hospital in order to keep you safe; in order for you to be alive for.

'The Stone in the Shoe'

> *Why do they (clients) need a social worker because we don't do things to people. We do things with people. So one of my colleagues put this really well: She says being a stone in the shoes and I really like that. That is possibly our role to be the stone in the shoe . . . And to be this stone in the shoe and say: Well hang on what about this? Is perhaps the most valuable stuff we can do. (Comment from a respondent)*

The social workers often described work with systems. There was a strong emphasis on working with client's family systems, and a concerted effort was made to work with other members of the team within a complex service system. In addition, there was the recurrent need to work across sector boundaries (which tended to be rigid), helping individual clients gain access to services while being conscious also of the organisational implications. Although they were working primarily with individuals and their families, these social workers tended to emphasise the need for change in systems from a social justice perspective, seeing it as a highly valued part of their role to be a 'stone in the shoe' always bringing people back to the possibilities for systemic change and how things might be done differently. This was typified by the following quote from a respondent:

> *From a social work perspective, how can I work this person into the system. (What are) its effects on the person, how can I help the system around and negotiate for them on their behalf.*

'Going Ten Rounds with the System'

This group of social workers was very conscious that their work was conducted in a secondary or host setting, where social work values, knowledge, and skills are not the dominant ones. Thus, they were aware that the very nature of much of their work was contested. As one put it, "you have to go ten rounds with the system to come to terms with which you are in that system." Although there was evidence that many of these expert social workers had considerable autonomy within their local agencies, they saw social work as being low in the interdisciplinary pecking order, "the least desired and [least] preferred" (as one respondent noted). Nevertheless, they demonstrated a continuing commitment to the struggle of doing good collaborative work firmly based in social work principles.

DISCUSSION

The present study has revealed that the dimensions of the professional expertise theory of Fook et al. (2000) were generally present at a high level in the sample of mental health social workers identified as experts by their peers. This suggests that the method of peer identification is effective as a means of identifying experts, and, second, it suggests that these mental health social workers are providing high-quality social work practice. We believe that they constitute a group from which there is much to learn that will be of value to educators, social work practitioners, and other mental health service providers.

What was striking with this sample was the considerable array of both substantive and procedural knowledge displayed by the respondents. These practitioners made use of a considerable amount of formal, theoretical knowledge, particularly from psychiatry. Many of the respondents exhibited knowledge of the substantive areas recommended by Sheehan and Ryan (2001) in their survey of mental health content in Bachelor of Social Work courses in Australian schools of social work. At the same time, they still clearly displayed transferability. This is "the ability to modify, change, and develop theory and knowledge so that it can be made readily relevant in different contexts" (Fook et al., 2000, p. 190). The utility and use of knowledge was very much contingent on its relevance and effectiveness for their practice.

The participants demonstrated a wide variety of skills. Whilst direct practice skills with clients were crucial, and were often paramount, in the situations they described, other skills were important such as advocacy skills, referring to and engaging other resources, and negotiating with other professions.

Creativity and flexibility were strongly featured. The ability to think laterally and creatively, to take the unexpected, but effective course of action was demonstrated by a number in the accounts. For example, when a social worker described taking a family to view a Christmas display at a department store, it was done in order to achieve a number of purposes: (1) as a means of providing an outlet for a family; (2) as a way of further assessing the mother's (the designated client) interaction with her children; and (3) as a method of moving the focus away from the mental health problem. The use of such a strategy was regarded as both bold and shocking by this respondent's colleagues.

In addition to the dimensions of expert practice identified by Fook et al. (2000), the present study identified six themes that are important in characterising expertise among this group of mental health social workers. They have acquired specialist knowledge on the job, which allows them to apply social work values, knowledge, and skills to mental health work with assurance (1). There was an impressive capacity to work consistently with 'the grind' of exceptionally demanding work (2). Reflecting on what the social workers said about this, it seems obvious that they are working in a traumatising environment, and are required to develop strategies for managing their own response to the trauma. What was striking about their strong passionate commitment to their clients was that they were able to use it to give purpose and energy to their actions, and that values were not divorced from knowledge and skill (3). They demonstrated the capacity to work at multiple levels simultaneously with cases that are already complex (4). In their description of work with individuals and families, they tended to refer to issues of social justice and maintained a focus on systemic change (5). It was an indication of their expertise that, within a host setting that they did not experience as being always supportive, they have continued to struggle, again and again with each particular client, to do good collaborative work from a clear social work perspective (6).

The extent to which these themes are stable features of expert social work in other settings requires further investigation. Some of them may be features of any professional work in the mental health field, and some may reflect the particular service system from which this sample was drawn.

The challenge for further professional education is to encourage flexibility, creativity, contextuality, and transferability within an environment of largely involuntary clients, statutory responsibilities, risk and dangerousness within mental health social work. It may be that much of our current "taken for granted" curriculum practices need to be reviewed in the context of these findings. For instance practice courses would necessarily have to include a focus on not only the principles of practice but also the particular adaptations required by practice in different fields. Similarly, field focussed content needs equally to give prominence to the specific practice potential of social work in particular contexts. Hence, educational programmes need to pay explicit attention to bringing together, on the one hand, social work values knowledge and skills and, on the other, the specific exigencies and demands of practice in a specific context such as mental health.

Specifically, this study demonstrates the benefits of engaging expert social workers as educators, in settings in which they are able to tell the story of their practice and give others the opportunity to use their experiences as a vehicle for critical reflection.

It is clear from this study that social workers in a demanding host mental health service system are able to put into effective practice identified features of social work expertise, and that it is not necessary to be reduced to the role of 'generic' mental health worker. Their specialist mental health knowledge and skill enhances rather than replaces their social work expertise. Indeed what does become clear is that these practitioners are primarily focussed on the personal, familial, occupational, and social dimensions of their clients' lives whilst continuing to hold a keen sense of the significance of the mental health policy and practice contexts. In this sense, these workers are exemplars of the service provision goals of the contemporary community-based mental health system in which almost all of the clients now live almost all of the time in the community, and the study clearly shows the central place that social work with its focus on social functioning can and should hold in such programs.

A note of caution needs to be considered about drawing too firm or full conclusions from this study. In particular it needs to be acknowledged that there are limitations inherent in some aspects of the methodology. The subjects are, for instance, drawn from only one urban Community Mental Health network and might not be representative of the population of mental health social workers from across the state or the country as a whole. However, the network is by far the largest provider of mental health services in the state and represents approximately one third of the whole urban area. A further source of possible limitations inherent in the study is the small sample size, which represents only about 1/6th of the population of mental health social workers in the network. The rationale and process for the choice of subjects has been previously explicated and the 'trade-off' is the gain in depth and quality of information that is potentially more available through the choice of a small sample size.

The chosen qualitative research methodology has borne considerable fruit. In the first place it has created a framework within which practitioners can readily and to good effect tell their practice "stories" which, given their deep and rich detail, provide a superb research and teaching resource material and a crucial example of the benefits of appreciating a broader understanding of evidence based approaches. In particular, the specific choice of using focus groups seems to have added considerably to the quality of the data as it provided a context for not only "hearing" the stories, but also of having them further developed and more fully explained through a process of peer expert interaction.

The work begun in this study will be developed by conducting 'observational interviews' of this sample of expert mental health social workers in their practice. 'Observational interviews' were utilised by Patricia Benner and her colleagues in studying critical care nurses and are a method in which workers are both observed and then asked questions about their actions and thoughts (Benner, Hooper-Kyriakidis, & Stannard, 1999). The present study will also be replicated in other countries for comparative purposes. This has already been done in Ireland and will shortly be done at a site in the United States of America. The authors will also be conducting a similar study with a group of expert paediatric social workers in Australia.

In conclusion, this study reaffirms the importance and uniqueness of social work in mental health. It also reinforces the importance of the knowledge, skills, and values exhibited by the expert social worker in this increasingly contested, risky, and dangerous practice environment.

REFERENCES

Benbenishty, R. (1992) 'An Overview of Methods to Elicit and Model Expert Clinical Judgment and Decision Making,' *Social Service Review*, 66(4), 598-616.

Benner, P., Hooper-Kyriakidis, P., & Stannard, D. (1999) *Clinical Wisdom and Intervention in Critical Care: A thinking-in-action approach*, Philadelphia, Saunders.

Campbell, J. (1996) 'Competence in Mental Health Social Work' in O'Hagen, K. (ed.) *Competence in Social Work Practice: A Practical Guide for Professionals*, London, Jessica Kingsley, pp. 70-85.

Dreyfus, H., & Dreyfus, S. (1986) Mind over Machine: The Power of Human Intuition and Expertise in the Era of the Computer, Oxford, Basil Blackwell.

Eraut, M. (1994) *Developing Professional Knowledge and Competence*, London, Falmer Press.

Fook, J., Ryan, M., & Hawkins, L. (1994) 'Becoming a Social Worker: Some educational implications from preliminary findings of a longitudinal study,' *Social Work Education*, 13(2), 5-26.

Fook, J., Ryan, M., & Hawkins, L. (1997a) 'Expert Social Work: An Exploratory Study,' *The Canadian Social Work Review*, 13(1), 7-22.

Fook, J., Ryan, M., & Hawkins, L. (1997b) 'Towards a Theory of Social Work Expertise,' *The British Journal of Social Work*, 27(2), 399-417.

Fook, J., Ryan, M., & Hawkins, L. (2000) *Professional Expertise: Practice, Theory, and Education for Working in Uncertainty*, London, Whiting & Birch.

Hawkins, L., Fook, J., & Ryan, M. (2001) 'Social Workers' Use of the Language of Social Justice,' *The British Journal of Social Work*, 31(1), 1-13.

Kellehear, A. (1993) *The Unobtrusive Researcher: A Guide to Methods*, Sydney, Allen, & Unwin.

Larson, M. (1990) 'In the matter of experts and professionals, or how possible is it to leave nothing unsaid,' in Torstendahl, R. & Burrage, M. (eds.) *The Formation of Professions*, London, Sage, pp. 24-50.

Leonard, P. (1998) *Postmodern Welfare*, London, Sage.

O'Hagen, K. (ed.) (1996) *Competence in Social Work Practice: A Practical Guide for Professionals*, London, Jessica Kingsley.

Ryan, M., Fook, J., & Hawkins, L. (1995) 'From Beginner to Graduate Social Worker: Preliminary findings of an Australian longitudinal study,' *The British Journal of Social Work*, 25(1), 17-35.

Sheehan, R., & Ryan, M. (2001) 'Educating for mental health practice: Results of a survey of mental health content in Bachelor of Social Work curricula in Australian schools of schools of social work,' *Social Work Education*, 20(3), 351-361.

Vass, A. (1996) *Social Work Competences: Core Knowledge, Values, and Skills*, London, Sage.

Wakefield, J. (1990) 'Expert systems, Socrates and the philosophy of mind' in Videka-Sherman, L., & Reid, W. (eds.) *Advances in Clinical Social Work Research*, Silver Springs, NASW Press, 92-100.

CROSSING BORDERS AT DIFFERENT LEVELS AND DIMENSIONS

Boundary-Spanning: An Ecological Reinterpretation of Social Work Practice in Health and Mental Health Systems

Toba Schwaber Kerson

SUMMARY. A boundary-spanning approach to practice traverses barriers to give social workers greater understanding of context, more latitude in interventions, and increased access to systems. This broad-based

Toba Schwaber Kerson, DSW, PhD, is Professor in the Graduate School of Social Work and Social Research at Bryn Mawr College. Professor Kerson is author of several books including *Social Work in Health Settings; Practice in Context* and *Boundary Spanning: An Ecological Reinterpretation of Social Work Practice in Health and Mental Health Systems.* She is on the editorial boards of several social work journals and is Book Review Editor for *Social Work in Health Care.*

Address correspondence to: Toba Schwaber Kerson, 925 Muirfield Road, Bryn Mawr, PA 19010-1920 (E-mail: tkerson@brynmawr.edu).

[Haworth co-indexing entry note]: "Boundary Spanning: An Ecological Reinterpretation of Social Work Practice in Health and Mental Health Systems." Kerson, Toba Schwaber. Co-published simultaneously in *Social Work in Mental Health* (The Haworth Social Work Practice Press, an imprint of The Haworth Press, Inc.) Vol. 2, No. 2/3, 2004, pp. 39-57; and: *Social Work Approaches in Health and Mental Health from Around the Globe* (ed: Metteri et al.) The Haworth Social Work Practice Press, an imprint of The Haworth Press, Inc., 2004, pp. 39-57. Single or multiple copies of this article are available for a fee from The Haworth Document Delivery Service [1-800-HAWORTH, 9:00 a.m. - 5:00 p.m. (EST). E-mail address: docdelivery@haworthpress.com].

approach helps social workers work in large, complex systems of care that demand more creativity and advocacy from practitioners in less time with less support. It draws from direct social work practice, program planning and management, social work administration, and business/organizational management. Spanned boundaries include those restricting knowledge bases and definitions of setting, those separating health from mental health, those that isolate systems of service delivery and levels and modalities of practice. *[Article copies available for a fee from The Haworth Document Delivery Service: 1-800-HAWORTH. E-mail address: <docdelivery@haworthpress.com> Website: <http://www.HaworthPress.com> © 2004 by The Haworth Press, Inc. All rights reserved.]*

KEYWORDS. Boundary-spanning, ecological perspective, social work practice approach

THE DEVELOPMENT OF THIS APPROACH TO PRACTICE

This addition to the ecological perspective was developed inductively, that is, it comes from the literature overlayed with my own practice experience and 28 years teaching practice, participating on social service organizations' advisory boards and keeping close touch with the work of many former students. As I tried to codify and articulate the perspective, and before I began to write, I gathered approximately 150 examples from social workers in a range of health and mental health settings so that the writing would take the shape of real practice. Examples were requested from the most creative social workers I knew including some who had redefined or stretched the boundaries of health-related activity. Each social worker was asked to provide a practice example involving:

1. relationships with two or more systems
2. managed care
3. the crossing of funding and/or policy boundaries
4. an ethical or another dilemma
5. an innovative assessment
6. creative or unusual intervention strategies
7. creative definition or social work roles, title, department, affiliation, or function, or
8. another dimension that is important for learning to be a social worker.

The simple form that followed asked for: the presenting problem, concern, or need, means of and tools used for assessment (including graphic and mapping devices), strategies and interventions (attach charts, pathways, timelines, or strategic plans), and conclusions. Several people sent examples of the closest they came to traditional social casework because they themselves did not classify what they were doing as social work. For example, one social worker organizes fund-raising events for self-help groups focused on a particular illness. I consider that all her activity (even organizing banquets) is on behalf of her population, and it is all health related. As a representative of an umbrella social services organization, another social worker scouts opportunities for new programming and new facilities in cities other than her own. Another manages all the step-down units in her hospital, while another manages a rehabilitation facility for substance abuse, and one is doing development work for her social work agency. All these activities are health-related and carried out on behalf of social work clientele.

I learned that social workers can be an extraordinarily persistent and patient lot. Many of the programs they describe were created over a long period while they were doing many other kinds of work in an organization. They held onto a vision, nurtured and tended it until it came to fruition. They all reported that managed care and the increasing attention to finances and financial constraints are extraordinarily frustrating and individual clients and consumers are moved too quickly through systems of care. Still, the social workers who remained positive and, indeed, upbeat about their work and their clients' possibilities were adaptive people who could maintain a clear, resolute realistic optimism. Thus, the conceptualization that follows comes from exposure to the writing of many disciplines, my teaching, and from the experiences of present and former students.

THE PLACE OF THIS APPROACH
IN AN ECOLOGICAL PERSPECTIVE

This approach is couched in an ecological perspective that was developed over many decades by Germain and Gitterman but informed by Meyer (1983, 1988) and many others beginning with Richmond in her work on case coordination and social diagnosis. Wakefield (1996a, 1996b), MacNair (1996), Gitterman and Shulman (1994), Allen-Meares and Lane (1987), Meyer (1983, 1988), Siporin (1980), and others have also made important contributions to this approach. For example, Karls and Wandrei (1994a, 1994b) developed the person-in-environment system (PIE) for describing, classifying, and coding adult social functioning problems, a fine contemporary effort to make an eco-logical perspective practical and systematic.

An ecological perspective is drawn from studies of ecology and general systems theory. General system theory has been described as a direction or program in the contemporary philosophy of science, an overarching frame-work, an abstract meta-theory, or a model of relationships between objects rather than a theory. The general systems paradigm provides social work with "a way of thinking and a means of organizing our perceptions of relat-edness and dynamic processes" (Ell and Northen, 1990:2). The framework purports that any systems–be they biological, social, or psychological–op-erate according to the same fundamental principles. All systems, for exam-ple, are open to influencing activity, are adaptive, incorporate notions of communication and control, have smaller organized activity flows that serve larger activity flows, and define the individual actor through the functional linking of subordinate parts to the operating whole. Systems are organized wholes consisting of elements that are related in varying nonlin-ear, mutual, or unidirectional and intermittent causal relationships. They are capable of primary and reactive change and evolution, and they main-tain differentiation through continuous input from and output to their envi-ronment. Thus systems are made up of complexes of interacting components or subsystems. Therefore, action flows within each system and outside of it, linking it to other systems and influencing that system.

The term ecological comes from ecology, the division of biology that stud-ies the relationships between organisms and all the parts of their environment that affect them and that they affect in any way. Ecology views people and their environments as interdependent. Individual components and aspects are separated for study in order to develop strategies for altering the relationships, but all units, dimensions, and aspects must be viewed together to be truly un-derstood. In biological terms, ecology deals with the relations between organ-isms and their environment. In sociological parlance, ecology is the branch concerned with the spacing of people and institutions and the resultant interde-pendency. Ecologists study adaptation to changes in the environment. Thus, studies of the relationship of structural, physical, and social stress to illness, life event research, and studies of social support and health are all part of an ecological understanding of the relationship of the individual to the environ-ment. "An ecosystemic perspective enlarges the unit of attention to include the individual, social institutions, culture, and the interactions and transactions among systems and within specific systems" (Ell and Northen, 1990:10). Thus an ecological perspective assumes a specific worldview and view of the individual from which all means of assessment, strategy building, and tools for intervention are drawn. I find an ecological perspective compatible with my own world view and view of the individual but not sufficiently applied or pragmatic for practicing or teaching the practice of social work. Therefore, I have added content from other disciplines and combined parts of the social work enterprise that have sometimes been seen as separate.

Like an ecological perspective, this boundary spanning approach is neither a model nor a theory but a useful way of thinking about practice (Meyer, 1988). A perspective is defined as the relationship of aspects of a subject to each other and to a whole as well as a mental view or outlook (American Heritage Dictionary of the English Language, 2000, p. 1311). The term perspective conveys depth and distance, as it does in art, lending added dimensions to understanding. A model is a description or representation of a structure that shows the proportions and arrangements of its component parts. A theory is "a scheme or system of ideas or statements held as an explanation or account for a group of facts or phenomena; a hypothesis that has been confirmed or established by observation or experiment and is propounded or accepted as accounting for the known facts; a statement of what are held to be the laws, principles or causes of something known or observed" (Oxford English Dictionary, 1971:278).

An ecological perspective presupposes the necessity of thinking systematically and necessarily disallows linearity. Thus, one cannot think in terms of one cause and one effect. It also presupposes that all systems have boundaries but that the boundaries are almost all permeable. In the case of social entities, that is, families, groups, organizations, or communities, boundaries can be redrawn or recast to work most effectively for the client. An ecological perspective is all about relationships, especially the relationship between people and their environments. It is particularly suited to social work practice because it is all encompassing and solves the perpetual social work dilemma of how to address the person and environment in a way that subsumes both. An ecological perspective suggests that clients, projects, programs, communities, and all the salient aspects of environment are parts of an interacting whole. In order to know why, when, and how to intervene, social workers must understand context, the interrelated conditions in which the client, project, program, or community exist.

General Systems Theory and Models of Business Management

Many frameworks for business management are derived from ecology and general systems theory as well. These frameworks have much to offer to social work practice. According to Drucker, with the exception of certain public health reforms, no new knowledge has contributed more to productivity and profitability in this century than developments in systems, people, and information management (Drucker, 1974, 1999). Specifically, business management frameworks provide pragmatic, clear ways for people to make sense of the structure, organization, and processes of systems. Because they are action-oriented and empowering, focused on the mission and goals of systems and the relationship of the work of all participants to the system, such frameworks undergird social workers' abilities to negotiate systems and advocate effectively for clients.

The ability to work within and manage these systems in highly productive, goal-oriented ways is critical for present and future social work practice. Such information has always been salient for social work practice, but the current environment in health and mental health care makes critical social workers' ability to understand organizations as systems, to speak the language and to maneuver in ways that help clients reach their goals (Levinson, 1992). In particular, the work of Peter Senge, Chris Argyris, John Kotter, Henry Mintzberg, and Peter Drucker informs this approach. Each of these people explores different dimensions of management that contribute to social workers' understanding of systems and to their ability to practice in increasingly complex environments. For example, Drucker's "management by objectives and control," Senge's "learning organizations," and Kotter's particular understanding of leadership can enrich social workers' understanding of systems, ecology, and an ecological perspective (Bailey and Grochau, 1993).

Drucker explains that every system that is more complicated than the simplest mechanical assemblage of inanimate matter contains multiple axes. Thus the body of every animal has many systems, including a skeletal-muscular system, several nervous systems, an ingestive/digestive/eliminating system, a respiratory system, sensory systems, and a reproductive system. While each system is to some degree autonomous, all interact, and each is an axis of organization. Organizations are not, and should not be, as complicated as biological organisms. Still, business and public service organizations must be constructed with several axes, including one for making decisions and distributing authority and information, as well as one for understanding the logic of the task and the dynamics of knowledge. In addition, individuals must have positions within these organizations so that they can understand and manage a number of axes related to tasks and assignments, decision responsibility, information, and relationships (Drucker, 1974:527).

Systems thinking is guided by two central principles. First, "structure influences behavior," which means that the ability to influence reality comes from recognizing structures that are controlling behavior and events. The second principle, "policy resistance," refers to the tendency of complex systems to resist efforts to change their behavior. Therefore, efforts to manipulate behavior will generally improve matters only in the short run and often lead to more problems in the long run (Senge, 1990:373-74). Such thinking uses systems archetypes to observe and fathom underlying structures in complex situations. For example, a mastery of systems thinking leads one to understand family problems or organization problems as emanating from underlying structures rather than from individual mistakes or negative intentions. Systems thinking leads to seeing "wholes" instead of "parts" and experiencing the interconnectedness of life. Thus, systems theory contributes to the understanding of organizations and management that has been developed in business, and social workers in health and mental health need this knowledge in order to be effective with and for their clients.

SOME BOUNDARIES TO BE SPANNED

Spanning Health and Mental Health

The first boundary that must be spanned is the one that separates health care from mental health care. New knowledge about the causes, symptoms, and treatment of a range of illnesses indicates that the dichotomy between physical health and mental health is false. While scientific and medical knowledge do not support this split, social responses, including administrative structures and funding streams, continue as if physical health and mental health were separate entities.

Expanding Definitions of Health-Related Settings

The second boundary area that must be redefined is the setting for health-related social work. The field can no longer afford to have factions fight from within about which settings are most prestigious or what are most acceptable. Definition of setting must be wherever populations are located whom we wish to help and where we can employ our knowledge and skills. Since the health-related social work moved from public health situations into university-affiliated hospital wards for indigent patients, we have created problems for and between ourselves. Certain historical moves seem overdrawn today, but it would be good if we could learn from them. For example, as psychiatry and psychoanalysis developed, social work established new boundaries in terms of setting and discipline, with psychiatric social work splitting off from medical social work. There was a time following that division when social workers set and allowed to be set for them parameters related to the levels of consciousness on which they could work. While psychiatrists could work on all levels, social workers could work only on the conscious and preconscious levels, never the unconscious level. At that time, many social workers worked one-on-one with their clients in fifty-minute increments, thus again setting tight parameters for their work and isolating themselves from the whole of the health-related enterprise. Today, social work practice in health and mental health occurs in schools, work sites, residential facilities, camps, homes, rehabilitation programs, neighborhood health centers, mental health centers, prisons, long-term care settings, advocacy and support groups, and hospitals.

Spanning Levels of Practice

A third boundary area exists between levels of practice. For many years, boundaries were drawn between modalities, with social workers calling themselves caseworkers, group workers, or community organizers. There were courses in schools of social work called "Group Work for Caseworkers" and "Community Organizing for Group Workers," but even within such courses, the lines were clear. The lines could sometimes be crossed, but the primary definition of the work was the tightly drawn modality. Now boundaries are drawn between those who are direct practitioners, those who do program development, and those who work in the policy arena. Those equally limiting barriers must be spanned for social work practitioners to act most effectively for and with clients.

Expanding Knowledge Bases

Other boundaries have been drawn through determining what kinds of knowledge bases could inform social work in health and mental health. The field has embraced, rejected, or debated various aspects of psychology, biology, sociology, economics, and political science, but sometimes has difficulty absorbing important knowledge that comes from sources not thought to reflect social work's value base. In the past, feuds erupted about the knowledge base for social work, such as that between the diagnostic and functional schools, or various schools of community action or group work. In the current managed care environment, the field has been loath to embrace the aspects of business management that might be very helpful to the social work enterprise. Many of these debates continue.

METHODS FOR SPANNING BOUNDARIES

This article briefly describes methods for social workers to span out-dated and limiting boundaries using: (1) population expertise; (2) mapping devices; (3) legal and ethical knowledge for better advocacy (Bertelli, 1998; Dickson, 1995; Sunley, 1997); (4) similar relationship skills for work with clients, colleagues, and organizations (Abramson, 1993; Gitterman & Shulman, 1994; Mulroy & Shay, 1997); (5) assessment techniques addressing individual, program, organizational, and community capacities (Griffiths, 1997; Kettner, Maroney, & Martin, 1999; Menefee, 1997; Saltz & Schaefer, 1996); (6) business management skills for understanding systems and the relationships within and between them (Drucker, 1999; Senge, 1990); and (7) multiple modes of intervention and evaluation (Mullen & Magnabasco, 1997; Zeira & Rosen, 1999).

Be population experts. Because it is not possible to know everything, yet one is measured in terms of knowledge and skill, health-related social workers can become expert only in terms of the knowledge and skill necessary to practice in relation to specific populations. That is, if one works with people with a chronic condition such as diabetes or schizophrenia, or a population such as mothers and young children or the very old, one must know the laws that entitle and restrict that population, understand the conditions themselves and possible medical and social interventions, the ways in which these conditions affect significant others, the ways that these conditions are handled in different cultures, etc.

Use mapping devices. Graphic representations or mapping devices are essential in this approach. Like other kinds of maps, these representations are meant to show social workers and clients/consumers where they are in a situation or in the work process, and to indicate direction for work. Turning something complex and overwhelming into a flat image on one page provides a sense of mastery and control if that image can suggest movement and direction. Varied use of such mapping devices allows social workers to span boundaries of time, place, and system in planning, monitoring, and evaluating their work.

Representations that have been found helpful are: organigraphs (Mintzberg, 1994; Mintzberg & Lampel, 1999; Mintzberg & Van der Heyden, 1999), driving forces maps (Christensen, 1997), balanced scorecards (Kaplan & Norton, 1996), and as well as genograms, ecomaps and systematic planned practice figures (Rosen, 1993; 1999). Visualizing complex sets of relationships and activities gives social workers a broader scope that deepens their understanding and helps them to choose points and methods of intervention (Tufte, 1997). These devices require that those who use them make their assumptions explicit through diagrams. They support contracting about how to view systems in context. Additionally, they provide ways to intensify moments in helping relationships by creating a concrete focus of attention. In all, such devices help social workers to assess, plan, make concrete, monitor, and compare. These devices can locate and follow social workers in their working systems, help them to visualize services for client systems, contribute to an understanding of organizations and systems and the relationships within and between them, and engage in strategic planning and programming. The organigraph, developed by Mintzberg and Van der Heyden (1999) to depict the workings of organizations, is one very helpful mapping device with which social workers may not yet be familiar. While traditional organizational charts seem to indicate that all units are independent boxes that are connected through chains of authority, the organigraph looks at how people and processes converge and where ideas flow. It maintains the conventional components of organizational chart (Figure 1): sets of people and machines and chains of command, and it adds two components: hubs and webs. In the hub, the process of managing brings together and coordinates the work of people who are intrinsically empowered. In the web, work is fluid and the facilitation of collaboration energizes the whole network. Social workers' ability to have adequate influence in their workplace and to be able to advocate for clients/consumers depends on their participation in hubs and webs.

Unlike ecomaps, genograms, or organizational charts, organigraphs often look very different from each other. Using the building materials of sets, chains, hubs, and webs, they assume the overall shape that presents the clearest portrait of an organization or system. The organigraph focuses on how processes and people come together and where ideas have to flow. It does not eliminate little boxes from organizational charts, but it introduces new components. The two conventional components in the device are sets of items (machines or people) and chains (assembly lines). The newer components are hubs and webs. In the hub, managing occurs at the center, bringing together and coordinating the work of people who are intrinsically empowered. In the

FIGURE 1. The Four Philosophies of Managing

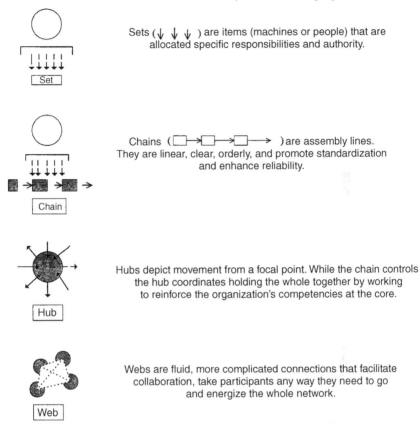

Sets (↓ ↓ ↓) are items (machines or people) that are allocated specific responsibilities and authority.

Chains (☐→☐→☐→) are assembly lines. They are linear, clear, orderly, and promote standardization and enhance reliability.

Hubs depict movement from a focal point. While the chain controls the hub coordinates holding the whole together by working to reinforce the organization's competencies at the core.

Webs are fluid, more complicated connections that facilitate collaboration, take participants any way they need to go and energize the whole network.

web, the work is fluid so that collaboration is facilitated and the whole network is energized.

Figure 2 is an example of an organigraph explained below. Because the hub, the Department of Case Management, is the center of the organigraph, the graphic resembles an ecomap. (For full discussion of the work that is illustrated here in the organigraph see Hammer and Kerson, 1998).

Figure 3 is another example of an organigraph that illustrates how several advocacy groups joined together and enlisted the media to influence their state legislature to reinstate funds for a critical program. (For full discussion of the work that is illustrated here, see Kerson, 2002.)

FIGURE 2. Department of Case Management at Fine Community Hospital

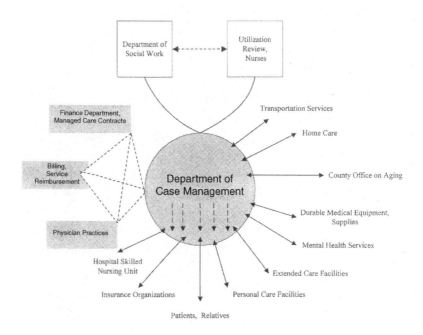

Understand legal and ethical realms. Understanding the legislation that affects particular populations will enable social workers to help clients use all the entitlements and protections available to them through state and federal government as well as the courts. A prime example in the United States is the Americans With Disabilities Act. The Americans With Disabilities Act (ADA) of 1990 is an important resource for those with physical and mental disabilities because it expands their rights, supports them as they become more fully participating members of society, and, most important, makes society responsible for accommodating the individual (Orlin, 1995). According to Orlin (1995:233), "The ADA establishes that the nation's goals regarding individuals with disabilities are to ensure equality of opportunity, full participation, independent living, and economic self-sufficiency." The ADA requires public accommodations and services, businesses, transportation, and communications authorities to treat people as if their disabilities do not matter while simultaneously requiring special treatment of them (Feldblum, 1991;

FIGURE 3. Options for Independence

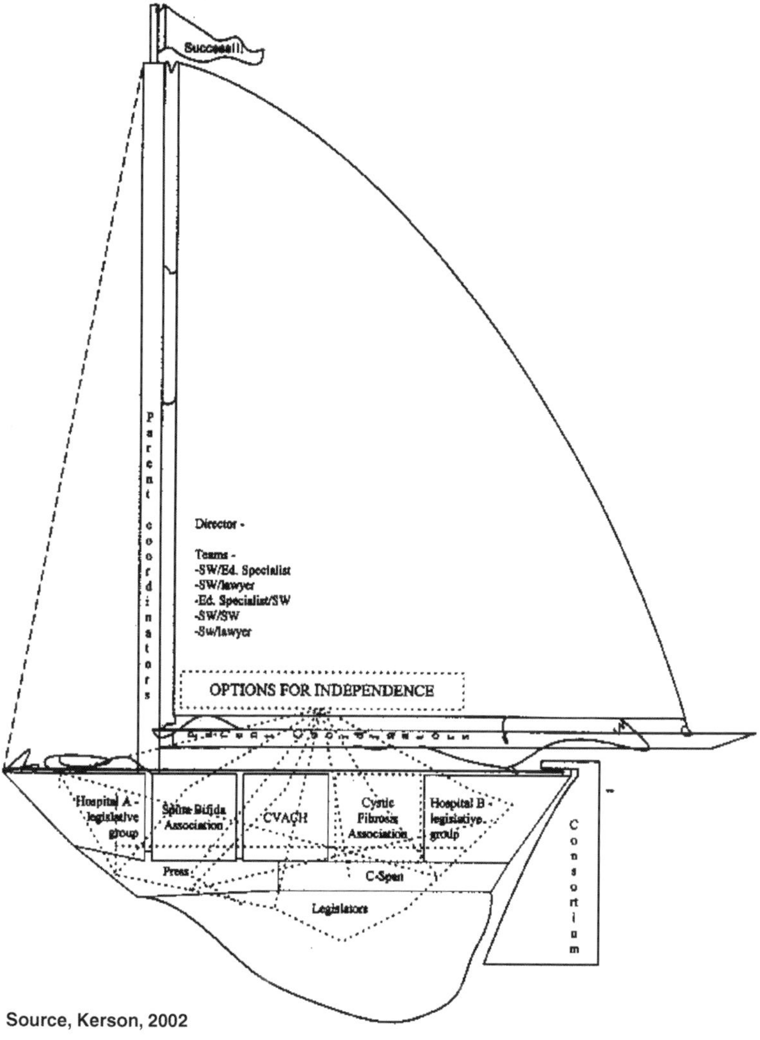

Source, Kerson, 2002

Kopels, 1995). Thus the ADA demands that society accommodate those with disabilities to the degree that will allow them to take their rightful places in society. More boundary-spanning opportunities are afforded by exploring and becoming comfortable with a range of ethical issues that are part of the work. Included here are ethical dilemmas that have no answer but that social workers must work within situations such as abortion, end of life decisions, and other medically and socially complex interventions. Examples of ethical decisions in which social workers might be involved include allocating limited health care resources, beginning or ending aggressive treatment, return to home or nursing home, and clashes between patient, family, and institutional interests.

Understand organizations, systems, linkages, and means of communication. This knowledge allows social workers to move more freely, build professional and interdisciplinary networks, understand patterns of authority and responsibility, and make organizations more responsive to clients and consumers. It reflects an ecological perspective because it assumes a constant interplay between the individual and the environment. Here issues are related to location, access, authority, and change; turf conflicts, teamwork and interdisciplinary, intra, and interagency work have to be managed. An overarching theme is that, although the settings where the work occurs may change, the critical importance of the work and the very high levels of knowledge and skill that social work requires will not. For example, because ill people are now hospitalized for as short a time as possible, work that used to occur in a hospital setting may now have to take place in a rehabilitation center, a nursing home, a senior center, in home care or a support group related to a specific illness or condition. Literature that supports this discussion of "place" is in social work administration, community and organizational development, and business.

Know that relationship skills are the same for everyone with whom you work. In this approach, excellent relationship skills are seen as a conduit for effecting change for the client system in every practice situation. Although both the context and strategies of the social worker in health care have become more extensive over the decades, the importance of the relationship between social worker and client system remains constant. No matter how large the unit of attention–whether it is a community, a large organization, a family, or an individual–the accomplishment of goals depends on the social worker's relationship abilities with individuals as clients or with individuals who represent larger client systems or health care organizations. Communication skills remain critical. The ability of social workers to understand the psychological nuances of relationship and to carry themselves differently in the relationship depending on the needs of the client system and the goals of the service are critical to this endeavor. It is argued that similar relationship skills are necessary for working with clients, colleagues, and those from all related systems. Therefore, traditional social work concepts such as self-awareness, conscious-use-of-self, and the overall capacity to develop and sustain relationships are explored. The overarching tasks of the relationship are to act as a conduit or catalyst for helping the client to reach goals, carry hope, lend a vision, and intervene in varied ways depending on the capacities and needs of the client system, the needs of other systems with whom social workers may be working, and the tasks necessary to meet needs and objectives. Such relationship skills are also critical in working in teams, in negotiating for clients with managed care and insurance company representatives, and with others with whom clients or social workers may have adversarial relationships. The notion of boundary spanning is essential to social workers' building and maintaining such relationships.

Use assessment across context as a continuous decision-making process. All practice concerns gathering information, making judgments and decisions, and acting on those judgments. The relationship of assessment to the development of objectives and outcome measures is critical for evaluation and continued support of individual client systems and programs. Whenever possible, practice must be empirically based, that is, closely linked to the products and processes of research. In relation to assessment, social workers must be able to answer the following questions: Who makes up the client/consumer system? What are the ecological boundaries that must be drawn to make sense of the situation? What are the probable parameters based on access, proximity, entitlement, and need that help the social worker to draw ecological boundaries? What range of services should be viewed as possible in this situation, especially in relation to the needs and capacities of the client system? What are the goals of the client/consumer seeking help? Are they realistic in the face of capacities and access? Are objectives drawn ahead of time by an organization, law, or funding source? What tools, such as mini mental status exams, activities of daily living scales, functional status, and community assessments, are available for assessment? Is the bio-psycho-social assessment sufficient to help client systems to develop strategies to reach their goals?

Understand two interventional sets. Two sets of interventions are seen as important for all social workers in health and mental health to master. The first set involves the planning process; determination of goals and objectives; uses and varieties of contracts in social work practice in health and mental health; the place, uses, and importance of strategizing; and the overarching importance of teamwork in all of social work practice. Typically, strategies are an amalgam of professional, family and other social supports, governmental, voluntary, self-help, relational, informational, and in-kind interventions. These may not occur at the same time or be carried out by one social worker, but the social worker is part of a large network of helpers moving in and out of work with the client system over time. Particular attention is paid to the relationship between self-help and professional help, as well as to interdisciplinary teamwork.

The second interventional set focuses on traditional direct practice tools. Here, advocacy is seen as an intervention in its own right, as well as part of all other interventions. Universal strategy issues include: the place of relationship techniques in all interventions, problem solving, the ability to partialize (to break down ways to address problems into small, manageable action steps), giving advice, the place of insight, interpretation and reflection, the use of questions designed to refocus the work (Are we working? What are we working on?), issues of timing (including sources of time constraints), court orders, funding sources, and varied models of intervention. Group strategies include work with individuals, families, organizations, and communities, in relating to other social workers, to interdisciplinary teams, and even in adversarial situations. Thus group techniques from problem solving, psychotherapy, and community work are important. In the same way, skills for developing and implementing policy help social workers understand, formulate and implement policies and remain active participants in policy debates. The usual boundaries are spanned in order to extend the panoply of interventions available to all health-related social workers.

Take an active part in all aspects of evaluation. The last part of this approach describes the relationship of the establishment of realistic goals and objectives to concrete measures of outcome to evaluate direct and indirect practice. Much of the discussion relates back to assessment, planning and contracting material, in ways that allow the objectives of the work to be measurable and thus possible to evaluate. Quality assurance and evaluation of social workers and their work are all dimensions of practice.

CONCLUSIONS

This discussion of the parts of this approach might suggest to the reader that learning is linear; that is, social workers use relationships to assess, then strategize, then intervene, then evaluate, all within a context that comprises history, laws, values, ethics, and organizational constraints. In fact, little learning or intervention is linear, and context is not made up of smaller and smaller concentric circles in which the social worker and client sit. Each element flows into all the others, and learning and intervening are both circular and continuous activities.

Overall, this boundary spanning approach is a next small step in the continued development of an ecological perspective for health-related social work. It combines management and more traditional social work information with a series of mapping devices, calls for social workers to be advocates and case managers, and requires excellent relationship skills and decision-making abilities. The approach is flexible and practical. Every part of the work is related to meeting the needs of clients, consumers, programs, and communities. The work answers these questions: What do clients need from me? What can they expect from me and from my profession here in my organization and in the larger systems to which they and I must relate? The work honors the past, is responsive to the present, and helps the social worker to proceed sensitively, professionally, and efficiently to help clients, consumers, programs, and communities enhance their well-being.

No approach to practice that has been developed so far is without serious flaws, and this reinterpretation is no exception. Overall, this is meant to broaden the scope of the social worker to incorporate more of the dimensions of context that are necessary for helping clients. Second, it encourages and enables social workers to act in powerful ways. It suggests that social workers must obtain and keep sufficient authority to do their work by becoming experts in relation to specific populations. It exhorts social workers to understand the needs and capacities of clients/consumers, programs, and communities, to understand the rich and complex systems in which the work occurs, and to use all possible levels of intervention to forward the work. All told, the purpose of boundary spanning is to enable social workers to span outmoded barriers to work as deeply and broadly as possible to help their clients reach their goals.

REFERENCES

Abramson, J. (1993). Orienting social work employees in interdisciplinary settings: Shaping professional and organizational perspectives. *Social Work*, 38(2) 152-157.

Allen-Meares, P. & Lane, B. (1987). Grounded social work practice in theory: Eco-systems. *Social Casework*, 68(9), 515-521.

Argyris, C. (1994). Good communication that blocks learning. *Harvard Business Review*. (July-August), 77-85.

Bailey, D. & Gorchau, K. E. (1993). Aligning leadership needs to the organizational state of development: Applying management theory to organizations. *Administration in Social Work*, 17(1), 23-28.

Bertelli, A. (1998). Should social workers engage in the unauthorized practice of law? *The Boston Public Interest Law Journal* 8(15): 1-28.

Bogdan, R. & Taylor, S. J. (1998). *Introduction to qualitative research methods: A guidebook & resource*. New York: John Wiley.

Christensen, C. M. (1997). Making strategy: Learning by doing. *Harvard Business Review* (November-December) 141-156.

Dickson, D. T. (1995). *Law in the health and human services: A guide for social workers, psychologists, psychiatrists, and related professionals*. New York: The Free Press.

Drucker, P. (1999). *Management challenges for the 21st century.* New York: Harper Business.

Feldblum, C. R. (1991). Employment protections. *Milbank Quarterly,* 69 (supp. 1-2), 81-110.

Germain, C. B. (1984). *Social work practice: An ecological perspective.* New York: Free Press.

Germain, C. B. & Gitterman, A. (1995). Ecological perspective. In R. L. Edwards (Ed.). *Encyclopedia of social work* (19th ed). (pp. 816-824). Washington, DC: NASW Press.

Gitterman, A. & Shulman, L. (1994). *Mutual aid groups, vulnerable populations, and the life cycle* (2nd ed.). New York: Columbia University Press.

Griffiths, L. (1997). Accomplishing team: Teamwork and categorization in two community mental health teams. *The Sociological Review,* 45(2), 59-78.

Hammer, D. L. & Kerson, T. S. (1998). Reducing the number of days for which insurers deny payment to the hospital: One primary objective for a newly configured department of case management. *Social Work in Health Care,* 28(2), 31.

Kaplan, R. S. & Norton, D. P. (1996). *The balanced scorecard: Translating strategy into action.* Boston, MA: Harvard Business School Press.

Karls, J. M. & Wandrei, K. E. (Eds.). (1994a). *Person-in-environment system: The PIE classification system for social functioning problems.* Washington, DC: NASW Press.

Karls, J. M. & Wandrei, K. E. (Eds.). (1994b). *PIE Manual: Person-in-environment system.* Washington, DC: NASW Press.

Kerson, T. S. (2002). *Boundary Spanning: An Ecological Reinterpretation of Social Work Practice in Health and Mental Health Systems.* New York: Columbia University Press.

Kettner, P. M., Maroney, R. M. & Martin, L. L. (1999). *Designing and managing programs: An effectiveness-based approach.* (2nd ed.). Thousand Oaks, CA: Sage.

Kopels, S. (1995). The Americans With Disabilities Act: A tool to combat poverty. *Journal of Social Work Education,* 31(3), 337-46.

MacNair, R. H. (1996). Theory for community practice in social work: The example of ecological community practice. *Journal of Community Practice* 3(3/4) 181-202.

McGoldrick, M. & Gerson, R. (1985). *Genograms in family assessment.* New York: W. W. Norton.

Menefee, D. (1997). Strategic administration of nonprofit human service organizations: A model for executive success in turbulent times. *Administration in Social Work,* 21(2), 1-19.

Meyer, C. (Ed.). (1983). *Clinical social work in the eco-systems perspective.* New York: Columbia University Press.

Meyer, C. (1988). The eco-systems perspective. In R. Dorfman (Ed.), *Paradigms of clinical social work* (pp. 275-94). New York: Brunner/Mazel.

Mintzberg, H. & Van der Heyden, L. (1999). Organigraphs: Drawing how companies really work. *Harvard Business Review* (September-October): 87-94.

Mullen, E. J. & Magnabosco, J. L. (1997). (Eds.). *Outcome measurement in the human services: Cross-cutting issues and methods* (pp. 3-19). Washington, DC: NASW Press.

Mulroy, E. A. & Shay, S. (1997). Nonprofit organizations and innovation: A model of neighborhood-based collaboration to prevent child maltreatment. *Social Work*, 42(5), 515-524.

Neugeboren, B. (1996). *Environmental practice in the human services: Integration of micro and macro roles, skills, and contexts.* New York: The Haworth Press, Inc.

Orlin, M. (1995). The Americans With Disabilities Act: Implications for social services. *Social Work*, 40(2), 233-39.

Rosen, A. (1993). Systematic planned practice. *Social Service Review*, 67(1), 84-100.

Rosen, A., Proctor, E. K. & Staudt, M. M. (1999). Social work research and the quest for effective practice. *Social Work Research*, 23(1), 4-14.

Saltz, C. C. & Schaefer, T. (1996). Interdisciplinary teams in health care: Integration of family caregivers. *Social Work in Health Care*, 22(3), 59-70.

Schatz, M. S., Jenkins, L. E. & Shaefor, B. W. (1990). Milford redefined: A model of generalist and advanced generalist social work. *Journal of Social Work Education*, 26: 217-31.

Senge, P. (1990). *The fifth discipline: The art and practice of the learning organization.* New York: Currency Doubleday.

Siporin, M. (1980). Ecological systems theory in social work. *Journal of Sociology and Social Welfare*, 7(4), 507-32.

Strauss, A. L. & Corbin, J. M. (1998). *Basics of qualitative research techniques & procedures for developing grounded theory* (2nd ed.). Thousand Oaks, CA: Sage.

Sunley, R. (1997). Advocacy in the new world of managed care. *Families in Society*, 78(1), 84-94.

Tufte, E. R. (1997). *Visual explanations: Images and quantities, evidence, and narrative.* Cheshire, CN: Graphics Press.

Wakefield, J. (1996a). Does social work need the eco-systems perspective? Pt. 1: Is the perspective clinically useful? *Social Service Review*, 70(1), 1-32.

Wakefield, J. (1996b). Does social work need the eco-systems perspective? Pt. 2: Does the perspective save social work from incoherence? *Social Service Review*, 70(2), 183-219.

Zeira, A. & Rosen, A. (1999). Intermediate outcomes pursued by practitioners: A Qualitative analysis. *Social Work Research* 23(2), 79-87.

Social Work Field Education as Social Development: A Lithuanian Case Study

Kathleen Tunney
Regina Kulys

SUMMARY. This article will discuss social development models and their application to the establishment of social work field education in Lithuania. A model of field education as social development is presented and discussed, with reference to promoting core social work knowledge, values and skills, establishing relationships between educational and social welfare institutions, and identifying the impact of field education programs on community well-being. Examples from the authors' experience in educational program development and implementation are presented, along with implications for international social work education. *[Article copies available for a fee from The Haworth Document Delivery Service: 1-800-HAWORTH. E-mail address: <docdelivery@haworthpress.com> Website: <http://www.HaworthPress.com> © 2004 by The Haworth Press, Inc. All rights reserved.]*

Kathleen Tunney, PhD, is Assistant Professor, Department of Social Work, Southern Illinois University Edwardsville, 1227 Peck Hall, Box 1450, Edwardsville, IL 62026 (E-mail: ktunney@siue.edu). Regina Kulys, PhD, is Associate Professor, Jane Addams College of Social Work, University of Illinois at Chicago, 1040 West Harrison, M/C 307, Chicago, IL 60607-7134 (E-mail: reginak@uic.edu).

Special thanks goes to Lucy Valciukas, for her passion, intelligence and hard work in developing the program and in sharing her reflections with us.

[Haworth co-indexing entry note]: "Social Work Field Education as Social Development: A Lithuanian Case Study." Tunney, Kathleen, and Regina Kulys. Co-published simultaneously in *Social Work in Mental Health* (The Haworth Social Work Practice Press, an imprint of The Haworth Press, Inc.) Vol. 2, No. 2/3, 2004, pp. 59-75; and: *Social Work Approaches in Health and Mental Health from Around the Globe* (ed: Metteri et al.) The Haworth Social Work Practice Press, an imprint of The Haworth Press, Inc., 2004, pp. 59-75. Single or multiple copies of this article are available for a fee from The Haworth Document Delivery Service [1-800-HAWORTH, 9:00 a.m. - 5:00 p.m. (EST). E-mail address: docdelivery@haworthpress.com].

Digital Object Identifier: 10.1300/J200v2n02_05

KEYWORDS. Social work practice, social work education, social development, international social work

INTRODUCTION

The purpose of this article is to examine the establishment of social work field education from the perspective of social development in a nation in which social work was a new profession and in which a strong network of community services did not exist. The article will trace the process of developing the field work component of social work education at the Centre for Social Welfare Professional Development at Vytautas Magnus University in Kaunas, Lithuania, from 1992 to 1997. Implications for social work education and practice in establishing new social work programs and working with community agencies will be presented.

The Centre for Social Welfare Professional Education (the Centre) was established in 1992 through a five-year grant from the National Conference of American Catholic Bishops. Besides being a prime mover in obtaining the grant, Sister Albina Pajarskaite, a founder of the Caritas chapter in Lithuania (an international Catholic Charities organization), provided additional support and inspiration as she saw the need for professionally trained social workers to meet the social welfare needs of a newly independent country. The overarching goal of the educational program was to "educate the educators"–to prepare future practitioners as educators to provide guidance and vision to the development of the social work profession in Lithuania. This was done by exposing the students to a variety of social work service delivery systems (Constable & Kulys, 1994; Constable & Mehta, 1994), through contributions from many countries, primarily the U.S. but also Poland, Australia, Canada, Ireland, Britain, and Germany. Three faculty from the U.S. were Fulbright scholars during the 1992-1997 period. At the very beginning of the program, the Centre offered only a master's degree, later extending to a baccalaureate degree. The Centre was administered by two co-directors who were social work educators at two different schools of social work in the United States. The second author was one of the co-directors.

Vytautaus Magnus University (VDU) was an essential partner in the development of the Centre, sanctioning a university-based education program leading to a masters degree. Faculty and staff of the Centre comprised existing faculty from VDU (in disciplines such as psychology and sociology) and existing university clerical staff members who were assigned to the Centre as support staff. Later, Centre graduates began to assume teaching and student supervision duties. Providing education through a diverse group of faculty was a particular strength of the program, in that it allowed a range of models of social work education and practice to be presented. The rationale for this educational focus was to enable students to make choices and create their own models of social work based on the needs of the country.

The Centre's educational program from the very beginning focused on social development, a crucial and deliberate choice given the acuity of social problems and the fragmentation of social welfare systems in Lithuania in the early 1990s shortly after its independence from the Soviet Union. While students were educated in knowledge, values, and skills of direct practice for work with vulnerable populations, the primary emphasis was always placed on assessing and intervening at multiple systems levels through program and community resource development, and on understanding the need for systems change and social action. In the second year, students were encouraged to engage in needs identification and program development in such areas as homelessness, school truancy and child neglect, among others.

Historically, social work education and practice have been criticized for over-emphasizing individual and family (micro level) problems and under-emphasizing the impact of culture, community, social injustice and economic inequity in the creation or exacerbation of individual problems (Bogo & Herington, 1986; Cox, 1995; Johnson, 1998; Mamphiswana & Noyoo, 2000; Ragab, 1990; Specht & Courtney, 1994). This individualistic emphasis has been seen as problematic both in Western countries and in other parts of the world, because it leaves students and practitioners ill-prepared to address larger systems issues and can lead to short-term solutions for long-term problems (Nimmagadda & Cowger, 1999). There is some evidence that the paradigm is changing in the direction of more community/locality development training, especially in nations newly independent such as South Africa or in Eastern/Central Europe, or in those who have experienced dramatic shifts in population health and density due to immigration and global economic shifts (Chui, Wong, & Chan, 1996; Gray & Simpson, 1998; Lusk & Stoesz, 1994; Murtaza, 1995; Taylor, 1999).

Because of the havoc wrought by the transition from a Soviet-run system to a democracy, social welfare services were underdeveloped in Lithuania with the result that many families and individuals were caught in a web of emerging social problems such as unemployment, poverty, crime, and lawlessness. The students' duties in their first year of field education focused on such skills as engagement/empathy, assessment, problem solving and linking to whatever resources were available. In the second year of the program, students usually continued in their first-year field practice settings, shifting their focus to applying basic social work skills of assessment and problem-solving to other systems levels. Several new community programs were created by Centre students and graduates in this manner; some of these programs will be discussed later in this paper.

The use of social development practice models as a framework for social work field education raises the question: What is meant by "social development"? Many different definitions exist. The next section of this paper will provide an overview of social development practice models, with a subsequent discussion of how these models apply to social work field education specifically (which has received less attention in the literature) and to the Centre's program.

CONCEPTUAL FRAMEWORKS:
MODELS OF SOCIAL DEVELOPMENT

The concept of social development is relatively new; after 50 years of its existence there is still little consensus concerning its key dimensions (Beverly & Sherraden, 1997; Jones, 1998; Midgley, 1997). Social development as a term began to be used after World War II, through the leadership of the United Nations, as societies struggled with reconstruction after the devastation of the war. The focus was on both social and economic development, and had philosophical roots in the utopian tradition that emphasizes the perfectibility of society. Another purpose of social development was to identify a role for government in the provision of social welfare services and social well-being (Specht & Courtney, 1994; Midgley, 1997).

Economic development and social development are different, yet overlapping concepts. Social development is more concerned with social justice, and the development and transformation of social structures to insure social justice (Tucker Rambally, 1999). Without an emphasis on social development, economic improvement can benefit different members of a society differentially, leaving some people behind, which can in turn lead to de-stabilization of a society and a widening income gap. Campfens (1996) for example states that the goal of social development, in contrast to economic development, is to promote the well-being of people.

Basic definitions of the concept of social development include the following: "the integrated, balanced, and unified development of society and the capacity of the social system to generate broad and favorable changes in levels of living . . . planned social change and economic development to promote the well-being of all. . . . Also embedded in the paradigm are . . . principles shared with social work, such as collaboration, cooperation, and social justice." (Tucker Rambally, 1999, p. 488). Social development is also defined as the process of working to link micro/macro level practice: "An encompassing concept that refers to a dual-focused holistic, system-ecologically oriented approach to seeking social advancement of individuals as well as broad scale societal institutions" (Asamoah, Healy, & Mayadas, 1997, p. 396).

Midgley (1995) defines social development as "a process of planned social change designed to promote the well-being of the population as a whole in conjunction with a dynamic process of economic development" (p. 23). Midgley contrasts social development with other approaches to social welfare such as philanthropy, social work, and social administration, because social development focuses primarily on developing communities as opposed to dealing with individuals through rehabilitative or service distribution approaches. It is of interest that Midgley appears to see social work as separate from social development while other authors have focused on the similarities. Midgley recognizes the degree to which social workers fall short of realizing the ideal of "social work as social development" because of a tendency to focus on micro level practice and on pathologies instead of strengths, an approach which can serve to isolate and enervate both workers and clients. Midgley (1993) suggests that social development strategies can be assessed in regard to their primary ideological foundations: beliefs about whether the most effective targets for social development interventions are located at the individual, governmental or locality level (individualist, collectivist, or populist ideologies). Regardless of ideology, Estes (1997) notes that "the ultimate goal of the social development movement, like that of the social work profession, is to secure for people everywhere the satisfaction of at least their basic social and material needs" (p. 45). The application of social development models to international social work practice and social work education is consistent with the focus of the social work profession on empowerment, social and economic justice, human rights, self-determination, access to resources and opportunities, and problem-solving with individuals, families, groups, and communities (International Federation of Social Workers, 2000; National Association of Social Workers, 1999).

Given the key importance of empowerment as a guiding principle for social work practice and education, social development models can be examined along a continuum of power and control. In essence, one dimension of social development is the degree to which different practice models assign expertise and decision making responsibility to various stakeholders in the development. For example, "outside expert" models assign the majority of control and expertise to the outside consultants; "partnership" models reflect greater equality and mutuality in control of resources and decision making between two or more entities in a development context; and "community-locality" models locate the majority of power, control of methods and goals, and expertise with local residents and stakeholders. Organizing social development approaches in this framework allows for an increased focus on decision making processes involved, which is useful in early program development, when securing maximum participation is a primary goal. These three basic approaches to social development practice will be briefly defined and discussed below, illustrated by examples from the Lithuanian educational program at the Centre.

Outside Expert Model: In this model of social development, the focus is more on "one-way" consultations which are often time-limited and issue-focused. The emphasis is on the outside expert giving advice and information to the consultees (Nimmagadda & Cowger, 1999). This approach was used in the Lithuanian Centre's program in the beginning when there was little social work expertise in the country. This meant that the social worker educators were "outsiders." While of necessity, this model was used early on, there were benefits and drawbacks. One benefit was that in Lithuania, outside experts were respected and assigned authority. This made it somewhat easier to introduce the idea of social work as a profession with its own areas of expertise. A drawback was that lodging the expertise in the outsiders tended to absolve the local participants from taking initiative to challenge the ideas if they did not fit the local reality. Under Communism, passivity was habit and a self-protective device. New conditions called for greater challenge to authority (even benign authority), but this was not initially forthcoming. Another drawback was that the social worker who was working as Field Coordinator did not have a PhD degree, which undermined her expert status with the university and made it harder for her to secure authority with the field agencies. As a skilled social work practitioner, however, she was able to use this identity as "outside expert" in her role with the students. She was *their* "outside expert," and could and did speak with authority in the seminars, while at the same time continually fostering autonomy among the students cum field supervisors.

Partnership Model: In this model, there is a greater emphasis on relationships among equals, in that two or more parties to the consultation on social development each have something to offer the others. There is an emphasis on resource and information exchange between the parties, for the mutual benefit of all. Benefits could be seen as financial, social, political or all of the above. While partnership models can be conceptualized as relationships between equals, this rarely occurs in international consultation practice, as the visitor often eclipses the local partners in regard to directing the process of social development (and therefore shaping the outcome). This is similar to the tendency of direct practitioners to direct the process of individual/family treatment, with less consideration for the desired goals of the client(s), even though social work values espouse a partnership model consistent with strengths-based approaches reflecting an egalitarian ideal (Watt, 1998).

In the Lithuanian educational program, use of a partnership model was a challenge because, at least in the beginning, there were no viable partners. The university accepted the program and granted it a Centre status, but within the university there was no one who wanted to "own" the program. Sister Pajarskaite, even though she had a doctorate, did not have it in the social sciences and was not a member of the university faculty. Thus the partners within the university had to be fostered and developed. The most relevant application of partnership strategies was in the ongoing negotiations with the university in regard to who would do what to make the program work. The university wanted something from the program: the educational status that came from being "on the cutting edge" of professional education in the region through support of social work as a new profession. The program wanted something from the university: the credibility that a university degree would give the students and the credibility of the social welfare services that they would ultimately create. The university provided ongoing support and was always willing to engage in discussion of program needs. The contractual component with the university clearly specified that the Centre would become the full responsibility of the university at the end of five years. This occurred in 1997 with the university assuming responsibility for the program.

Community-Locality Model: This model focuses on people-centered development, involving key stakeholders at every stage of the process to identify social problems, options, resources and solutions that could have applications beyond the locality (Jones, 1998; Rothman, 2000). Nayaran (2000) quotes Cox (1998) who defines social development as "people-centered development which rests on five foundations: awareness-raising; social mobilization, participation, self-reliance, and sustainability" (Narayan, p. 195). Estes (1997) and Lusk and Stoesz (1994) suggest that social development can best be described as locality-based with links to a larger social development picture. In other words, the process of social development identifies a social problem on a local level (neighborhood, community) and seeks to involve key stakeholders in a response to the problem, which can be attempted within the parameters of local resources and within the control of those affected by the problem at the local level, which in turn can build coalitions for addressing larger social problems that may have contributed to the local problems. In essence, this approach reflects a "developmental" approach to social development, with local issues addressed before, or along with, state or national issues.

A challenge to locality development in the establishment of field education programs is offered by Tucker Rambally (1999): "In order to have field education, there must be a field. In developed countries where social work education is well established, there exists a network of agencies and trained social workers to provide the practicum. However, in some developing countries . . . the field has to be established, and there is an arguably expanded role for field education in promoting organizational change and social development" (p. 485). Rambally discusses the role of the university in providing leadership to agencies in developing program initiatives in Barbados. While agency-university partnerships are not unknown in social work, the emphasis on social development as opposed to case work as well as the leadership role assumed by the field division in the university distinguishes this innovation from the more traditional models of collaboration. The emphasis in these models of field education is on the empowerment and resource development of the agencies themselves, thereby increasing their ability to better serve clients and to educate students in field practice. This again illustrates the "locality development" approach to social development.

The goal of the Centre was to move from outside expert models to community-locality development models, such that the local educational and practice community would have full ownership of educational and community programs. In order to achieve this goal, it was necessary to conceptualize the whole system of stakeholders, creating a "map" of the components of the system which could assist in selectively applying the social development models as needed. That model is presented and discussed in the next section.

A MODEL OF FIELD EDUCATION AS SOCIAL DEVELOPMENT

In order to understand the complex interrelationships between social work field education and community development, the authors developed the following model involving four interrelated components: (1) Core social work professional knowledge, values, and skills; (2) Educational program development and student skill development; (3) Agency-service development among field placement agencies; and, (4) Impact on the community as a result of the educational program's contribution to service development (see Figure 1). Following a brief description of the overall model, each component will be separately discussed, using examples from the Centre's program as illustration.

The model has a primary direction that traces a developmental path: The first step is the identification of a basic set of social work knowledge, skills and values to be offered through the university system. From there, field agencies are introduced to the university program through students, faculty and field instructors together developing field placements and collaborating on creating agency programs that can provide mutual benefits to student, agency, and improved client/community well-being. Lessons learned from the community can, in turn, contribute to the further clarification of social work knowledge, skills, and val-

FIGURE 1. A Model of Field Education as a Social Development

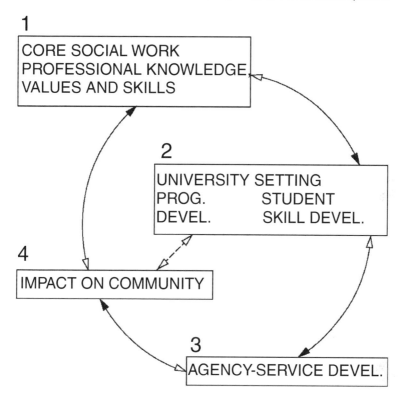

ues for practice which have demonstrated relevance to local needs and conditions.

While the model in Figure 1 describes the basic direction, it also accounts for the realities of practice through the use of bi-directional arrows, showing that the developmental influences are not only one-way. For example, the agencies also influenced the university, in that the agencies identified additional educational needs of the students. Also, the community impacted the agencies, in pinpointing the need for preparation and joint planning. Further, the community influenced the university by the positive recognition that Centre students and graduates were accorded for their work, which reflected positively on the university. And ultimately the community helped to shape the definition of core knowledge, values, and skills of social work as a result of the students' and graduates' increasing ability to use problem solving and advocacy skills within both the university and agency settings.

Core Social Work Knowledge, Values, and Skills: The Centre program utilized a range of theoretical perspectives to provide a "starter set" of concepts that students were encouraged to question, modify and shape according to the degree to which these perspectives were useful in describing and explaining human behavior in the current environmental context. Some of these approaches that were considered core knowledge included ecological systems theory, human life course development, family systems theories, community and policy analysis frameworks, and social development models. Social work values were emphasized in the program, particularly those related to human rights and dignity, social justice, access to resources and social change. It should be noted that the term "social change" is a value-neutral term–social change can be either helpful or harmful. The Centre faculty and students strove to be part of healthy growth and social change, to stem the tide of social change resulting in social disorganization, which occurred when the Soviet system of social welfare services (however minimal) broke down. Social work skills such as engagement, assessment, and problem solving were taught with the emphasis on application of these skills across systems levels.

Field education in community agencies was seen as the most effective means of skill development. This emphasis on field education as most important among a variety of experiential learning methods was one of the factors that made the Centre's program at VDU unique among other social work programs in Lithuania that developed around the same time. In essence, basic social work knowledge, values, and skills were applied directly to field setting, serving the program goal of social development, which also helped to foster a "common vocabulary" with social workers in other nations. Students were encouraged to build on the common core to create service models reflecting local needs and respecting local culture. Focus groups with students suggest that these goals were met; students participating in the groups reported that core values, concepts and processes of social work were being provided in the context of a collegial model of education and practice (Watt, 1998).

University Setting and Student Skill Development: Because of the Centre's emphasis on establishing social work as a new profession in Lithuania, an important component of the social development process was the establishment of the program within the university setting. Since typically in Eastern Europe, professional programs existed outside the university setting, an early challenge was establishing the credibility of the program within the university, including the importance of field experience as a part of the university degree. A later challenge in program development was sustaining the quality of the social work program in light of increasing demands, including the increasing numbers of students wanting a social work education. This demand later led to the creation of a baccalaureate program in social work at the Vytautas Magnus

University. More students meant more need for field placements and field supervisors in order to uphold the program goal of providing meaningful community-based practice experiences for students.

In regard to student skill development, skills of direct practice were taught in classroom and field, along with community assessment, program development and supervision skills. Methods of instruction (outside of formal classes) included three weekly field seminars–one for first-year students, which focused on direct practice dilemmas and strategies; one for second-year students, which focused on program development and collaboration models; and one for field instructors, which focused on skills for student supervision. The seminars were co-led by visiting faculty (including the first author of this article) and by the Coordinator of Field Practica, a Lithuanian-Australian funded through the United Nations Development Project (UNDP) for a two-year period specifically to develop field education and other community-based social work initiatives (Valciukas, 1996). Visiting faculty and the Field Coordinator also provided direct supervision of students within agencies, as well as inservice education and liaison services to agencies' staff and administrators on their request.

Challenges in student skill development included the overwhelming volume of human need, compared to resource availability; agency and student expectations for positive changes were easily and often frustrated. Issues of autonomy, power, and boundary setting were also encountered, in that students were often seen as "lowest on the totem pole," particularly in the mental health settings, yet paradoxically were charged with responsibility of "making miracles" for severely impaired patients. Another issue that arose (again, particularly in medical and mental health settings) was that of role conflict and role competition. For example, nurses often felt that the social workers' new functions usurped some of their own job responsibilities; they felt threatened about displacement from their desperately needed jobs. This is consistent with conflicts in the West in regard to a fight for professional identity in high-pressure settings such as managed care.

Advocacy for human rights and dignity was another challenge for the Centre's social work students. Many agency employees had not been exposed to the social work professional value system that emphasized treating clients and families with dignity and respect, without regard to their behavior or characteristics of mental illness, substance abuse, or single-parent status. Attitudes encountered by the students were punitive at worst and paternalistic at best, requiring students to articulate professional values and ethics that they were only just learning, and which in some cases conflicted with their own personal value systems. Another major challenge encountered in the placements and discussed a great deal in the seminars was the pressure to "do something, do anything" to respond to client needs and agency demands. Seminar leaders strove to help students and field instructors develop a "reflective practitioner" identity, in order to not exacerbate a bad situation with a knee-jerk response, but this was difficult when the spotlight was on them; they had a need to see themselves (and be seen) as effective and helpful. Working step-by-step through a case study in a "group supervision" model was helpful for group support and problem solving. It also assisted in the development of local "teaching cases" for future generations of students and supervisors who would attend the ongoing seminars. The Field Coordinator utilized strategies such as sending students into field placements "two by two," so that each would have a built-in support in an often intrusive system. The Field Coordinator would encourage students to work for "little breakthroughs," and emphasized the importance of "working alongside" them wherever possible, letting them observe her, but also watching "from a distance" as they worked with individuals and families and negotiated for more resources. The Field Coordinator said ". . . they need their own process . . . I had a different kind of confidence, and they needed to develop their own . . . [they] needed to know that the supervisor wouldn't always be there." She, too, was overwhelmed by the "chasm of knowledge gap"; as a result, she developed the strategy of letting the students ask questions and tell her what they needed to know. She had no reservations about sharing her expertise, but was highly attuned to the need to generate skills and confidence in the students as quickly as possible.

Agency-Services Development: Along with the communication of social development concepts in the field seminars, a related question is: How was the idea of social development communicated to field agencies? First, agency administrators were approached; it was made clear that they were in charge of assigning tasks; students were there to serve the agency and to learn about the agency's needs and challenges. The university supervisor would be in charge of teaching students to apply classroom theories to field issues, while making special efforts to include the agency supervisor in all phases of the placement, including creation of learning goals, progress toward goals and agency needs for particular services. Students often became employees after graduation, because the agencies saw the students as supportive of the agency's goals and dilemmas, without having a motive of "tearing down" the agency. The purpose of the field seminars was to integrate the realities of practice with the concepts of classroom education, which was especially difficult when this classroom education was offered (in the beginning) in the English language by Western educators with little familiarity with these aforementioned realities of practice.

So, in essence, the students were teachers–teachers of the field agencies and classroom faculty in regard to the social development needs that they saw in their agency field sites. This reflected an interesting set of role reversals, and often, delicate negotiations of role and expertise when everyone was trying to figure out what they had to offer each other. This was particularly challenging in a culture where the concept of "expert" was both powerful and rapidly changing, due to the influx of Westerners with knowledge and money to apply to a variety of enterprises, including social welfare and higher education.

Another dimension of social development in the Lithuania program was reflected in the collaborative relationships forged between religious, educational, and civil authorities to develop resources where none existed before. Sister Albina was a prime mover in the early years in the agreements made between municipalities, CARITAS, with the students actively involved in designing programs with the assistance of faculty. These students later became field supervisors and/or directors in the new agencies that they helped to create.

Key issues here also included the importance of identifying and resolving conflicts over duties and expectations as openly as possible (a challenge in and of itself, due to the Soviet legacy of secrecy and mistrust). Therefore, communication skills on the part of faculty, liaisons, and students were a key component of the social development strategy. Introducing the concept of collaborative work was also a challenge, again in part due to the necessity under the Soviet system to conceal information and ideas as opposed to openly sharing them. One benefit in the early days was that many of the first students had been professionals in other fields such as medicine, architecture, nursing or teaching, and so had professional and political skills that were useful in making the transition to social work and social welfare programs. Another useful strategy (consistent with the partnership models of social development) was that agency personnel were invited to participate as co-trainers in some of the regional training events sponsored by the university Centre's faculty.

For example, one visiting professor with expertise in child welfare would routinely include as co-presenters in his community training courses child welfare agency employees who demonstrated a clear understanding of children's needs and creative approaches to scarcity and resource development. This training was designed and implemented with the direct involvement of agency staff and students, thereby providing social development in the form of learning how to communicate information to a professional audience. This strategy reflects the key importance of partnerships on a "micro" level. A presentation team of three people (faculty, agency, and student) can be seen as a microcosm of social development and a model for cooperation in larger groupings. Thus, the Centre took a lead role in providing training, which grew out of collaboration.

Key themes in agency-service development could be described under the heading of "starting small and sustaining relationships," consistent with the locality development approach to social development: listening to staff at all levels, linking to basic resources of the university and community, creating resources in collaboration with staff, and formalizing these collaborations into discrete training and service programs wherever possible.

Impact on Community: Consistent with the emphasis on outcomes assessment, which is becoming increasingly important in achieving credibility for social work education and practice in the West, the Centre engaged in an ongoing effort to evaluate its accomplishments and establish directions for the future. At this writing, over 100 Master of Social Work students have graduated and are working in community-based programs. Many of these programs are those the graduates themselves created during their student days. For example, the Family Centre, a program of CARITAS, was largely staffed by students from its inception and continues to offer innovative services to children and families. Other graduates developed a youth shelter program as students, which continues to provide services today. A residential program for elderly men and women as well as young single mothers and their children is called "Kartu Namai" (Generation House). This is another example of a community-based program partially financed by the municipality that began with the students of the Centre, supported by the university and by visiting and local faculty.

In keeping with the Centre's original purpose of "educating the educators," by 2002 four alumni of the Centre have been awarded PhD degrees, and four others are in the process of completing their PhD education. Many graduates are engaged in teaching, research, public service, and curriculum development at Vytautas Magnus University as well as other institutions of higher education in Lithuania. Further, the university-community partnership mode has been successfully sustained, resulting in ongoing training on a range of social welfare and community leadership development topics. Several graduates obtained grants from foundations such as the Soros Open Society Fund to provide in-service education to community workers engaged in the provision of services to various groups of people such as the elderly.

CONCLUSIONS AND IMPLICATIONS

Based on the authors' experiences in social work education in Lithuania, it can be concluded that social development is a useful conceptual framework for establishing social work field education. This approach: (1) keeps all components of the system in view–providing a "map"; (2) reinforces the importance of exchange and empowerment among all components, recognizing the dynamic and changing relationships among the stakeholders in development; (3) serves as a teaching tool, guiding students in understanding relationships between systems; and, (4) emphasizes the larger goal: making an impact on the community through professional education and professional services that are locally-derived and locally-sustained.

Taking the analysis one step further, thinking of social work field education as social development could change the way we implement field education in developing countries. Indeed, this same conceptualization could change the way we implement field education everywhere–including cities or regions within Western countries where individual and community development has stalled due to long-term poverty, short-term economic fluctuations, and changes in social welfare policy priorities.

What might change if we apply a social development model to field education? Field education programs would: (1) reflect greater balance between building students' skills in direct practice with skills for advocacy and community coalition building; (2) recruit new sites for student placement that can offer students opportunities to participate in program development, implementation, and evaluation, with social work supervision being provided "off-site" if necessary; and, (3) recognize the importance of multiple stakeholders in making field education work, expanding the scope of influence of social work programs beyond the traditional social service agency setting.

An eloquent call for linking social work and social development, which is supported by the experience of the authors, is made by Taylor (1997). This statement challenges the profession of social work to re-examine its main value to the societies of the future:

> Social work education has, with its generic (and eclectic) focus, attempted to educate social workers to fulfil therapeutic, regulatory, advocacy, and social change and reform functions. This all-encompassing approach has failed to educate social work students to fulfill any of these functions adequately. . . . Social work must choose a more limited focus [on] training for social development: more concretely, one in which community development, self-help and mutual aid activities are central. . . . To this end, curricula would concentrate on providing, among other things, knowledge of social policy development and the skills of animation, conscientization, and empowerment on a community level. (p. 316-317)

In summary, field education can be seen as "more than a medium for the integration of knowledge and values . . . [it] can act as a force for organizational change and a catalyst for social development" (Tucker Rambally,

1999, p. 494). In order to implement effectively social work field education as a force for change, the skills of social development need to be defined and operationalized for use by students, agency field supervisors and university liaison staff. This process of applying social development concepts can be a powerful translation and transformation of the familiar social work knowledge, skills, and values such as self-determination, strengths identification, and resource development.

REFERENCES

Asamoah, Y., Kealy, L., & Mayadas, N. (1997). Ending the international-domestic dichotomy: New approaches to a global curriculum for the millennium. *Journal of Social Work Education, 33*, 389-401.

Beverly, S., & Sherraden, M. (1986). Investment in human development as a social development strategy. *Social Development Issues, 19*, 1-18.

Bogo, M., & Herington, W. (1986). Field instruction based on a social development practice model: The example of Sri Lanka. *International Social Work, 29*, 73-82.

Campfens, H. (1996). Partnerships in international development: Evolution in practice and concept. *International Social Work, 39*, 201-223.

Chui, W., Wong, Y., & Chan, C. (1996). Social work education for social development. *Journal of Applied Social Sciences, 21*, 15-25.

Constable, R., & Kulys, R. (1994). *Field education in developing nations*. Chicago: Lyceum Books.

Constable, R., & Mehta, V. (1994). *Education for social work in Eastern Europe: Changing horizons*. Chicago: Lyceum Books.

Cox, D.R. (1995). Social development and social work education: The USA's continuing leadership in a changing world. *Social Development Issues, 17*, 1-18.

Estes, R.J. (1997). Social work, social development, and community welfare centers in international perspective. *International Social Work, 40*, 43-55.

Gray, M., & Simpson, B. (1998). Developmental social work education: A field example. *International Social Work, 41*, 227-237.

International Federation of Social Workers. (2000). *Definition of social work*. Berne, Switzerland: Author.

Johnson, A.K. (1998). The revitalization of community practice: Characteristics, competencies, and curricula for community-based services. *Journal of Community Practice, 5*, 37-62.

Jones, J.F. (1998). From globe to village: Understanding local social development. *Social Development Issues, 20*, 1-16.

Lusk, M.W., & Stoesz, D. (1994). International social work in a global economy. *Journal of Multicultural Social Work, 3*, 101-113.

Mamphiswana, D., & Noyoo, N. (2000). Social work education in a changing socio-political and economic dispensation: Perspectives from South Africa. *International Social Work, 43*, 21-32.

Midgley, J. (1993). Ideological roots of social development strategies. *Social Development Issues, 15*, 1-13.

Midgley, J. (1995). *Social development: The development perspective in social welfare*. Thousand Oaks, CA: Sage.

Midgley, J. (1997). International and comparative social welfare. In R. Blank (Ed.), *Encyclopedia of Social Work* (19th ed.), pp. 1490-1520. Washington, DC: NASW Press.

Murtaza, N. (1995). The social development paradigm in Third World countries: Unfulfilled promise. *Social Development Issues, 17*, 57-65.

Narayan, L. (2000). Freire and Gandhi: Their relevance for social work education. *International Social Work, 43*, 193-204.

National Association of Social Workers. (1999). *NASW code of ethics*. Alexandria, VA: Author.

Nimmagadda, J., & Cowger, C. (1999). Cross-cultural practice: Social worker ingenuity in the indigenization of practice knowledge. *International Social Work, 42*, 261-276.

Ragab, I.A. (1990). How social work can take root in developing countries. *Social Development Issues, 12*, 38-51.

Rothman, J. (2000). Collaborative self-help community development: When is the strategy warranted? *Journal of Community Practice, 7*, 89-105.

Specht, H., & Courtney, P. (1994). *Unfaithful angels: How social work has abandoned its mission*. New York: The Free Press.

Taylor, Z. (1999). Values, theories, and methods in social work education: A culturally transferable core? *International Social Work, 42*, 309-318.

Tucker Rambally, R.E. (1999). Field education in a developing country: Promoting organizational change and social development. *International Social Work, 42*, 485-496.

Valciukas, L. (1996). *Report to the United Nations Development Project*. Kaunas, Lithuania: UNDP Newsletter.

Watt, J.W. (1998). Social work education in the Baltic states and Poland: Students assess their programs. *International Social Work, 41*, 103-113.

Outcomes Measurement:
A Social Work Framework for Health
and Mental Health Policy and Practice

Edward J. Mullen

SUMMARY. Outcomes measurement in health and mental health should be of vital concern to social workers since public support and financing will follow evidence of effectiveness. Social work in health and mental health requires a framework for conceptualizing outcomes measurement so that the profession can focus clearly on the work to be done in outcomes measurement. This framework should distinguish among the various ways that outcomes measurement can be used to advance policy, program and practice. This article discusses two applications of outcomes measurement, namely for improving policies and programs, and, second, for conducting outcomes research. Other dimensions that could be included in an outcomes measurement framework for social work in health and mental health are identified but not elaborated. The author's objective is to make a strong case for the role that outcomes measurement can play in both the improvement of social work policies

Edward J. Mullen, BS, MSW, DSW, is Willma and Albert Musher Chair Professor, Columbia University School of Social Work, 622 West 113th Street, New York, NY 10025 (E-mail: ejm3@columbia.edu).

The assistance of Gretchen Borges, Haluk Soydan, Lawrence Martin, David Menefee, Karun Singh, James Dumpson, Chito Trillana, and Gerald Hanley in the preparation of this paper is acknowledged.

[Haworth co-indexing entry note]: "Outcomes Measurement: A Social Work Framework for Health and Mental Health Policy and Practice." Mullen, Edward J. Co-published simultaneously in *Social Work in Mental Health* (The Haworth Social Work Practice Press, an imprint of The Haworth Press, Inc.) Vol. 2, No. 2/3, 2004, pp. 77-93; and: *Social Work Approaches in Health and Mental Health from Around the Globe* (ed: Metteri et al.) The Haworth Social Work Practice Press, an imprint of The Haworth Press, Inc., 2004, pp. 77-93. Single or multiple copies of this article are available for a fee from The Haworth Document Delivery Service [1-800-HAWORTH, 9:00 a.m. - 5:00 p.m. (EST). E-mail address: docdelivery@haworthpress.com].

and programs in health care, through performance measurement, as well as in advancing the healthcare knowledge base, through outcomes research. *[Article copies available for a fee from The Haworth Document Delivery Service: 1-800-HAWORTH. E-mail address: <docdelivery@haworthpress.com> Website: <http://www.HaworthPress.com> © 2004 by The Haworth Press, Inc. All rights reserved.]*

KEYWORDS. Outcomes measurement, outcomes research, performance measurement, comparative performance measurement, health, mental health

This article examines measurement of social work outcomes in health and mental health. Outcomes measurement is the systematic, empirical observation of the effects of social programs on the achievement of objectives having to do with improving the health and mental health of individuals and populations. Outcomes measurement plays an important role in both the improvement of social work policies and programs, through performance measurement, as well as in advancing knowledge about how to provide effective and efficient social services in health and mental health, through outcomes research. Outcomes measurement in health and mental health is of vital concern to social workers since evidence of effectiveness is required for public support and financing.

Concern with cost-containment is ever present. But in addition to cost-containment, purchasers and payers of health care as well as some health care providers are expecting quality and evidence of desired outcomes from care provided. Payers no longer accept the argument that increased funding will improve quality and outcomes. At one time, health care professionals including social workers may have enjoyed public confidence regarding the effectiveness of their interventions but that is no longer the case. Rather, the assumption now is that there is room for improvement in performance. Public confidence has shifted to public skepticism. Consumers and payers now expect professionals to provide evidence of effectiveness, responsiveness to expectations, and fairness in financial burden. In response to these widespread expectations health care systems are shifting rapidly toward performance measurement and management with a focus on outcomes. Calls for evidence-based practice, practice guidelines, and best value are ever present. In the coming years these efforts will intensify. Each of the health care professions, including social work, will be challenged to provide evidence regarding their respective contributions to health care system performance. Social work in health and mental health will be expected to articulate the specific contributions the profession can make to health system goal attainment and to provide evidence that health system outcomes are measurably improved because of social work interventions.

SOCIAL WORK NEEDS AN OUTCOMES FRAMEWORK

Social work is vulnerable because it lacks a conceptual framework for defining specifications of the profession's outcomes in health care and for clearly focusing on the work to be done in outcomes measurement. If social work is to address the demand that its contribution to health care be documented, the social work community needs to engage in discourse regarding how to conceptualize the intended outcomes of its interventions; what criteria can be used to indicate attainment of those objectives; and, how to measure those outcomes. This framework must specify social work's particular contribution to health care, consistent with health system goals set by broader constituencies. Social workers must develop a common language for talking about objectives and outcomes in health care. A common outcomes language is required for effective communication between social work practitioners themselves as well as for clear communication among practitioners, managers, policy analysts, and researchers both within the profession and across professions. The profession's outcomes framework needs to be inclusive of the range of interventions that contribute to health system performance, from policy to direct practice interventions, and cutting across system levels, from neighborhoods to nations. Defining such a framework presents a significant challenge since social workers in health and mental health are deeply involved in efforts to improve the health status and care of whole populations–internationally, nationally, and locally–as well as with efforts to improve outcomes for individuals and families at the clinical level.

A number of outcomes related conceptual frameworks currently exist in health and mental health that social work can draw from in specification of social work outcomes. For example, the Australian National Health Information Management Group Working Party on Health Outcomes and Priorities developed an outcomes indicator framework that can be applied to specific health conditions and population groups (Australia Institute of Health and Welfare and Commonwealth Department of Health and Family Services, 1997). A similar framework has been developed by Statistics Canada and the Canadian Institute for Health Information (2001) in their Health Indicators project. Mrazek and Haggert (1994) outline a useful framework for considering mental health outcomes pertaining to prevention. Nevertheless, many of these frameworks are specific to a particular national context or a specific aspect of health or mental health. Most importantly, they are silent regarding social work's specific contributions to health and mental health outcomes.

Some argue against an outcomes measurement framework specific to social work. Critics say that health and mental health outcomes frameworks should be general, cutting across professional contributions. However, while social work shares many objectives with other health care professionals, social work does have special objectives and special emphases that need to be made explicit by framing objectives as well as outcomes indicators pertaining to those objectives. For example, whereas medical professionals may stress outcomes pertaining to disease states and outcomes indicators such as physiologic measures, social work is focused on quality of life objectives and outcomes. Most importantly, there is great confusion in practice as well as in the literature about social work's objectives, intended outcomes, and ways of demonstrating the attainment of outcomes in health and mental health care. This confusion undermines the profession's capacity to speak clearly and convincingly about its contributions. Accordingly, the profession needs to establish some common understanding about objectives and outcomes, and this requires a broad conceptual framework as well as specialized frameworks applicable to specific areas of social work practice.

WHAT IS OUTCOMES MEASUREMENT?

Although the topic of outcomes measurement attracts considerable attention in many countries, there is confusion regarding what is meant by the phrase "outcomes measurement." A common language pertaining to "outcomes" and "outcomes measurement" is missing. Moreover, as a profession, social workers lack a common understanding of why we engage in outcomes measurement. As noted recently by Maloney and Chaiken (1999, p. 3): "An outcomes vocabulary has emerged in health care. However, there is no consensus to date on the best approach to defining and measuring outcomes." They continue, "Without a precise translation of the word outcome in its application to health care, outcome means different things to different people." They observe that "the definition used by one organization or person can vary significantly from that used by other groups or individuals. Most often outcomes are categorized according to the perspective of the users of the data" They cite differences among such users as managed care organizations (e.g., focusing on cost-effective service indicators), accrediting organizations (e.g., screening for early detection), clinicians (e.g., clinical results), and patients (e.g., health improvement, functional status, quality of life).

Donabedian (1981) defined health outcomes as changes in a patient's current and future health status that can be attributed to antecedent health care. This definition is widely accepted within healthcare. In the report *Australia's Health 2000*, health outcome is defined as "A health related change due to a preventive or clinical intervention or service. (The intervention may be single or multiple and the outcome may relate to a person, group or population or be partly or wholly due to the intervention)" (Australia Institute of Health and Welfare, 2000, p. 444). The British National Health Service describes outcomes as "The attributable effect of an intervention or its lack on a previous health state" (United Kingdom Clearing House on Health Outcomes, March 1997). Definitions of "outcomes" applicable to general public sector services are consistent with these health definitions. In the United States, the Government Performance and Results Act of 1993 (1993, §1115) defines outcome as "the results of a program activity compared to its intended purpose." All of these references tie outcomes to identifiable, traceable interventions, at least in part.

ORIGINS OF OUTCOMES MEASUREMENT IN HEALTH CARE

Elsewhere we have reviewed the origins of outcomes measurement in the human services (Mullen & Magnabosco, 1997). In health care the interest in outcomes measurement was stimulated in the early 1980s when studies of health care interventions documented great variation in the use of specific types of medical interventions among practitioners, and that little was known about what caused the variation or the effectiveness of the interventions. As noted by the Agency for Healthcare Research and Quality (2000, §2):

> researchers discovered that 'geography is destiny.' Time and again, studies documented that medical practices as commonplace as hysterectomy and hernia repair were performed much more frequently in some areas than in others, even when there were no differences in the underlying rates of disease. Furthermore, there was often no information about the end results for the patients who received a particular procedure, and few comparative studies to show which interventions were most effective.

In response to the recognition that evidence of effectiveness was lacking and wide variation existed in practice, it has now become widely accepted that outcomes measurement can be of benefit: (1) to clinicians and patients by providing evidence of benefits, risks, and results of interventions so that they are able to make more informed decisions; and (2) to health care managers and purchasers, by providing information regarding effective interventions that can be used to improve the quality and value of health care (Agency for Healthcare Research and Quality, March 2000). The widespread emphasis on public accountability has moved outcomes measurement in many countries into the forefront. As noted by the Australia Institute of Health and Welfare and Commonwealth Department of Health and Family Services (1997, p. 3) concerning national health priority areas:

> A changing focus of accountability in government, from inputs (for example, total expenditure) to outputs and outcomes, has led to an increasing emphasis on the measurement of activities and the impact that these activities have. In the health sector, this has seen a general shift in emphasis from a focus on service providers and inputs, to a system also incorporating a focus on outcomes and the consumer.

DIMENSIONS OF A SOCIAL WORK HEALTH AND MENTAL HEALTH OUTCOMES MEASUREMENT FRAMEWORK

In the following I outline dimensions to be included in a health and mental health social work outcomes measurement framework. Such a framework should provide for outcomes measurement variation by: (1) system level; (2) geographical unit; (3) outcomes measurement questions asked; (4) effects sought across a continuum of possibilities; and (5) purpose of the outcomes measurement program.

System Level

An outcomes framework should distinguish among system levels. Here the question is "What level of intervention is being examined?" In health care there are at least three levels: (1) clinical level involving outcomes of clinical interventions with specific individuals; (2) program level involving outcomes of a program or a program component on a population or a sample of a population; (3) system level involving outcomes of a health care system on a population or a sample of a population.

Geographical Unit

Geographical unit can further classify system level outcomes with possible units being: (1) local community or neighborhood, in which questions would address outcomes of a health system program on community residents; (2) municipality, in which questions would address health program outcomes on a municipality's population or subpopulation; (3) state, province, region or the like, in which questions would focus on even larger population aggregates; (4) nation in the case of questions regarding national health system outcomes; and (5) sets of nations, such as health system outcomes on World Health Organization or Organization for Economic Co-operation and Development member nations.

Question Asked

This outcomes measurement dimension pertains to the questions asked. There are at least five types of question: (1) efficacy–what are the outcomes, as measured under highly controlled conditions–the ability of health care, at its best, to improve the patient's well-being and the degree to which this is achieved; (2) effectiveness–what are the outcomes, as measured in routine practice; (3) efficiency–what are the greatest outcomes at the lowest costs; (4) quality–how good are the outcomes, as compared to some standard of desirability; (5) equity–how fair are the outcomes, as distributed across groups according to some view of what is a fair share of benefits and burdens.

Of particular importance to a social work outcomes framework are questions of effectiveness and equity. Efficacy refers to outcomes examined in controlled trials removed from practice contexts, but effectiveness refers to outcomes found in the context of real world applications, the settings in which social workers function. Oftentimes what is found to be effective in controlled trials is found to be ineffective in natural settings unless additional environmental modifications are made. Social work has a special skill in addressing effectiveness questions involving real world applications. And, with social work's commitment to social justice, equity questions are directly relevant at all system levels.

Effects

Five types of effects relevant to health and mental health are described by Clancy and Eisenberg (1998): (1) mortality (e.g., infant death rate); (2) physiologic (e.g., blood pressure); (3) clinical events (e.g., stroke); (4) generic or specific health related quality of life measures of symptoms (e.g., difficulty breathing), of function (e.g., social adjustment or adaptation), and, of care experience (e.g., consumer survey); and (5) composite measures of outcomes and time (e.g., quality-adjusted life years; potential years of life lost; disability adjusted life years; health-adjusted life expectancy). This is a particularly important dimension for social work in health care. As noted by Clancy and Eisenberg (1998, pp. 245-6):

Clinical success has traditionally been appraised in terms of mortality, physiological measures such as blood pressure or diagnostic test results that are surrogates for physiologic function (such as laboratory tests, radiographic findings, or biopsy results), and definable clinical events. Clinical trials have produced these objective measures as their primary dependent variables. Seldom have patients' preferences for outcomes and risks of treatment been used to evaluate health services; they often have been perceived as important but subjective and unreliable. However, patients and clinicians must increasingly make decisions associated with different types of outcomes, such as length of survival, preservation of function, or pain relief.

Of special importance to social work Clancy and Eisenberg observe:

> The dimensions of health and well-being that encompass consequences for the daily lives of individual patients are referred to as health-related quality of life (HRQL). Broad aspects of HRQL include health perceptions, symptoms, functioning, and patients' preferences and values. The sum of these constitutes a continuum of effects of health care services on health and well-being, ranging from mortality to patient satisfaction.

Social workers have special expertise and interest in measures of health related quality of life, such as symptoms, functional measures, and experiences with care including satisfaction and access. Mortality measures and composite measures, which address life quality as well as length of life, are of special pertinence to the formation of social work policy. Social work has special sensitivity to measures that take into account the preferences and perspectives of clients.

Purposes of Outcome Measurements

There are two equally important but very different purposes for doing outcomes measurement. The first is to support performance measurement and management. The second is to conduct outcomes research. Confusion has resulted when these differences of purpose have been ignored in outcomes measurement practice and in the literature.

Outcomes Research as a Purpose of Outcomes Measurement

Outcomes measurement can serve the purpose of outcomes research. In health care, outcomes research, like performance measurement, has as its purpose improving the quality of interventions and policies governing interventions. In outcomes research, applied social science research methods are typically used to enhance the validity of causal assertions regarding measured associations between interventions and outcomes, whereas such methods may be less important in performance measurement. Outcomes research is conducted, not to improve the performance of individual programs directly, but rather to contribute to general knowledge about health care intervention outcomes. Consequently, with increased understanding of what works, policies and programs can be improved.

The Agency for Healthcare Research and Quality (March 2000, § 1) has defined outcomes research as:

> Outcomes research seeks to understand the end results of particular health care practices and interventions. End results include effects that people experience and care about, such as change in the ability to function. In particular, for individuals with chronic conditions–where cure is not always possible–end results include quality of life as well as mortality. By linking the care people get to the outcomes they experience, outcomes research has become the key to developing better ways to monitor and improve the quality of care.

Two types of outcomes research are important in health care. One focuses on efficacy and effectiveness studies, which seek to establish the effects of specific health care interventions using social science research methods. The product of this line of research is seen in what is now called "evidence-based practice" and "practice guidelines." The second type of outcomes research in health care is the study of social indicators, but only when social indicators are used to assess and monitor health system performance at the population level. Also of importance is a third type of outcomes research, namely methodological research, which aims to develop measures for use in subsequent outcomes research.

Methodological research–developing measures. Methodological research aimed at developing measuring instruments has resulted in the production of a large number of measures that can be used in both outcomes research and performance measurement. These measures are readily available in print (e.g., Murphy, Plake, Impara, Spies, & Buros Institute of Mental Measures, 2002) and on the Web (e.g., Agency for Healthcare Research and Quality, 1997). This area of outcomes research has been very productive yet much more needs to be done, especially pertaining to measures that are sensitive to cultural variations, consumer expectations and preferences, and quality of life measures.

Efficacy and effectiveness research. Outcomes research examining the efficacy and effectiveness of specific health care interventions has received considerable attention both in social work and in health care for some time. During the past two decades this area of research has been unusually productive. Accordingly, information regarding the effectiveness of a wide range of healthcare interventions is now readily available and much of this information is easily accessible on the Web (e.g., Cochrane Collaboration, 2002). The Cochrane Collaboration has established a library available on the Web that provides over one thousand systematic research syntheses (reviews) and over 800 protocols (proposed reviews in preparation) encompassing a large spectrum of health and mental health intervention and disease areas. The recently formed Campbell Collaboration, which is modeled on the Cochrane Collaboration, is especially relevant since it focuses on social work and social welfare intervention effectiveness research (as well as education and criminal justice research). A global network of Cochrane and Campbell collaborators is contributing to a database of randomized controlled trials and controlled clinical trials (C2-SPECTR) which now contains approximately 11,000 studies.

It is remarkable how productive this area of outcomes research has been in the last decade. Whereas no clear evidence was available about social work intervention effectiveness when my colleagues and I examined this in the early 1970s, much information is now available for use by policy makers, managers, clinicians, and consumers alike (Mullen, Dumpson, & Associates, 1972). Perhaps because the evidence has mounted so recently, little has yet found its way into everyday practice (Mullen & Bacon, 2002). Accordingly, transfer of this evidenced-based practice knowledge into clinical settings and into policy is a high priority.

Policy research and monitoring. Social indicators research designed to monitor health and mental health status as well as trends in status is an increasing significant type of outcomes research. The intent of this research is to inform policy as well as program decisions and directions. Social indicators research conducted to examine the effects of health care policies or programs on populations is a powerful application of outcomes research methods. Many outcomes measurement efforts at local, national, and international levels now include such policy research efforts under the rubric of outcomes measurement. For example, the framework of health indicators for outcome-oriented policy making developed in the 1999 Occasional Paper issued by the Organisation for Economic Co-operation and Development (OECD) on health outcomes in OECD countries includes social indicators in its definition of outcomes research. The OECD report states: "Given that the primary objective of health policy is to improve the health status in a population, health status indicators are included under the umbrella of health outcomes to describe the level of health and the variations across countries and over time" (Jee & Or, 1999, p. 12).

The OECD framework identifies outcome-oriented policy-making health indicators for four measures of health status: (1) mortality (e.g., life expectancy, infant mortality, standardized causes of mortality rates, premature mortality–potential years of life lost); (2) general and disease specific morbidity and quality of life (e.g., perceived health status; measures of impairment, disability, and handicap; multi-dimensional health status measures such as the SF-36, EuroQol, and Health Utility Index; prevalence and incidence of specific diseases); (3) composite health measures of mortality and morbidity (e.g., disability-free life expectancy; health-adjusted life expectancy; disability-adjusted life years).

Another example of social indicators health research is found in the human development reports issued annually since 1990 by the United Nations Development Programme (UNDP). The *Human Development Report 2000* uses four composite indices to measure different dimensions of human development, which are of significance to health and mental health (Human Development Index, Gender-Related Development Index, Human Poverty Index for Developing Countries; Human Poverty Index for Industrialized Countries). As noted in the UNDP report, "tracking changes in outcomes is the focus of the human development indices" (United Nations Development Programme, 2000, p. 99). To assess the adequacy of progress in achieving outcomes the report calls for benchmarking so that countries set specific, time-bound targets for making progress toward achieving publicly stated outcome goals. This is an excellent example of using outcomes measurement for policy research purposes.

Performance Measurement

Outcomes measurement is used to measure the performance of single programs or systems, not comparing the performance with that of other programs or systems. Also, outcomes measurement can be used to compare program or system performance with other programs or systems of like kind.

Non-comparative performance measurement. Outcomes measurement is widely used in both the public and private sectors to examine the performance of individual health and mental health systems and programs. The information resulting from performance measurement is used for system and program improvement. Performance measurement typically includes the regular collection and reporting of information about the efficiency, quality, and effectiveness of programs. The widespread use of performance measurement, especially in public sector programs, marks a shift from the traditional focus on inputs or resources used and processes or program activities, to outcomes, or what is being accomplished. Martin and Kettner (1996) outline a comprehensive performance measurement model in which outcomes are key to what are called effectiveness measures, by which effectiveness is defined as the ratio of results, accomplishments, or impacts (outcomes) to resources consumed (inputs) as measured by cost per outcome, outcomes per full-time-equivalent employee, and outcomes per hour worked. As noted by Martin and Kettner, outcomes measurement for assessing program performance is rapidly becoming the expectation in governmental agencies and publicly funded programs. For example, in the United States the Government Performance and Results Act of 1993 now requires that all federal departments report effectiveness (outcomes) performance data to Congress as part of the annual budget process. This legislation requires that all federal agencies set specific outcome objectives, identify outcomes indicators pertaining to those objectives, measure achievement of outcomes, and report results. It is expected that these results will then be used to set new objectives in a continuous year-to-year process of improvement.

When used in performance measurement, outcomes measurement is usually incorporated into a continuous quality improvement process. Performance frameworks incorporating outcomes measurement have been promulgated for some time by organizations such as the European Foundation for Quality Management. The Foundation's EFQM Excellence Model (© EFQM) places results and outcomes measurement center stage. The model is promulgated by a number of European governments. For instance, in the United Kingdom Cabinet report "Getting It Together: A Guide to Public Schemes and the Delivery of Public Services" (United Kingdom Cabinet Report, 2000) the EFQM model is explicitly promoted for public sector organizations as part of the Modernizing Government programme. This report presents a comprehensive guide to quality schemes relevant to public sector policies and programs with particular reference to health and education. The report promotes other quality schemes as well, including Investors in People, Charter Mark, and ISO 9000. These schemes are promoted as a way to help the public sector deliver Modernizing Government policy, including improved outcomes.

Another example of the use of outcomes measurement to assess performance is illustrated in the report of the Organization for Economic Co-Operation and Development (OECD) examining performance measurement in OECD country health systems (Hurst & Jee-Hughes, 2001). The OECD paper places outcomes measurement at the center of the performance measurement and management cycle. This cycle begins with the health care system and an assumption that improvements in this system are desired. In the next phase in the cycle, conceptualization, and measurement of performance including outcomes, specific intended outcomes would be identified and outcomes indicators would be specified for measurement. The third phase is an analysis of the outcomes indicator data that is collected and comparison of the data with intended objectives. Action to improve the health system based on the analysis of performance data is the final step in the cycle. The OECD paper defines health system performance as the extent to which the system is meeting established objectives.

The OECD report notes:

> There is mounting pressure on health systems to improve their performance. Technological advances and rising consumer expectations continue to raise demand. There is also growing concern about medical errors. Meanwhile, both public and private funders continue to strive to contain costs and control supply. Consequently, there is an intensification of the search for improvement in value for money. . . . The result is widespread interest in the explicit measurement of the 'performance' of health systems, embracing quality, efficiency, and equity goals and in influencing or managing performance. (Hurst & Jee-Hughes, 2001, p. 8)

According to the OECD report twelve member countries are developing performance frameworks and indicators for the country's health care systems.

Comparative performance measurement. Typically performance measurement schemes are used to examine how well a program is doing relative to some internal criteria, such as baseline performance, or in relation to a desired level of performance. Outcomes measurement can also be used in a process of comparative performance measurement (CPM). In CPM the questions are: "How well is a program performing relative to other similar programs?"; "Is a program's performance among the best of its kind or among the worst of its kind?" CPM can be used to identify which programs are among the best of their kind, and, in doing so, suggest best practices. As noted in an Urban Institute report, when applied to public sector and non-profit organizations such comparisons increase competition for limited resources and clientele (Morley, Bryant, & Hatry, 2001).

An example of comparative performance assessment in health and mental health is the United Kingdom's Best Value program (United Kingdom Office of the Deputy Prime Minister, 2002). In the United Kingdom comparative performance assessment is an integral component of the national Modernizing Government initiative. The UK's Best Value regime, a part of that initiative that is applicable to all parts of local government, requires that local councils compare their performance with other similar councils. In health and social services, local authorities are required to measure and report on Best Value outcomes, that is, established performance targets and national standards. The Best Value program mandates that local councils seek continuous improvement in services with respect to cost and outcomes; disseminate Best Value performance plans for public comment; and implement regular performance reviews to raise standards and reduce costs. The UK National Health Service Plan stipulates that comparative performance improvement be supported by a new system of targets and incentives (United Kingdom National Health Service, 2000).

A second example of comparative performance measurement in the public sector is the Comparative Performance Measurement Program of the International City/County Management Association (ICMA) based in Canada and the United States (International City/County Management Association, 2002). Through this program, the ICMA assists local governments in measuring, comparing, and improving municipal service delivery. In keeping with the goals of comparative performance measurement, this program provides a means for local governments to share data on a range of programs, benchmark their performance to comparable jurisdictions, and improve service delivery through the application of best management practices and efficient use of resources.

An important example of comparative performance assessment is found in the World Health Organization (WHO) publication "The World Health Report 2000." This report assesses and compares national health system performance among its 191 member countries. A number of performance measures are used to report on each country's absolute performance. The WHO report argues that it is achievement relative to resources that is the critical measure of a health system's performance. By matching countries with similar resources allocated to healthcare, the WHO calculates potential. In addressing the question of how well health systems perform, the WHO report states:

> Assessing how well a health system does its job requires dealing with two large questions. The first is how to measure the outcomes of interest–that is, to determine what is achieved with respect to the three objectives of good health, responsiveness, and fair financial contribution (attainment). The second is how to compare those attainments with what the system should be able to accomplish–that is, the best that could be achieved with the same resources (performance). (p. 23)

Accordingly, to assess relative performance the WHO calculated an upper limit or performance "frontier," corresponding to the most that could be expected of a health system. As the report notes:

> This frontier–derived using information from many countries but with a specific value for each country–represents the level of attainment which a health system might achieve, but which no country surpasses. At the

other extreme, a lower boundary needs to be defined for the least that could be demanded of the health system. With this scale it is possible to see how much of this potential has been realized. In other words, comparing actual attainment with potential shows how far from its own frontier of maximal performance is each country's health system. (p. 41)

Comparative performance assessment is a powerful use of outcomes measurement. It is through comparison that explanations for important differences in performance emerge. For example, because of the comparative approach taken in the WHO analysis, the authors were able to draw the following conclusion:

This report asserts that the differing degrees of efficiency with which health systems organize and finance themselves, and react to the needs of their populations, explain much of the widening gap in death rates between the rich and poor, in countries and between countries, around the world. Even among countries with similar income levels, there are unacceptably large variations in health outcomes. The report finds that inequalities in life expectancy persist, and are strongly associated with socioeconomic class, even in countries that enjoy an average of quite good health. Furthermore the gap between rich and poor widens when life expectancy is divided into years in good health and years of disability. In effect, the poor not only have shorter lives than the non-poor, (but) a bigger part of their lifetime is surrendered to disability. (p. 2)

CONCLUSION

Social work has an important contribution to make to the performance of health systems worldwide, a contribution at all system levels, ranging from clinical services to policy and system shaping at national and international levels. However, documentation of those contributions is required. At the clinical level the profession must move rapidly toward evidence based practice models (Mullen, 2002a & 2002b), adopting practice guidelines that have empirical support (Mullen & Bacon, 2002), derived from outcomes research. Social work research can contribute to the development of validated practice guidelines and system and policy relevant indicator systems. Outcomes measurement, guided by clearly articulated conceptual frameworks, can strengthen social works' voice in health and mental health care. A framework oriented to social work outcomes should highlight the specific contributions that the profession intends to make to individuals, families, and communities–in addition to its contributions to system performance and knowledge development. These outcomes can be planned in partnership with other health and mental health care stakeholders, including potential recipients of care. A clearly defined framework will enhance our ability to communicate about outcomes with clarity. Transparency of objectives and intended outcomes will strengthen the profession's position in increasingly skeptical national debates about best value in health and mental health.

My purpose has been to urge the social work profession to adopt an outcomes-oriented view. I have said that an outcomes-oriented approach to social work policy and practice is necessary if the profession is to make the contribution to health and mental health that it has the potential to make. However, I have concluded that we cannot move toward an outcomes-oriented approach unless we think clearly about what we mean by outcomes, and how outcomes can be measured, so that the data gathered is relevant to social work purposes. I have argued for a conceptual framework pertaining to outcomes measurement in social work in health and mental health that incorporates four key dimensions: the purpose for conducting outcomes measurement; the system level wherein outcomes measurement is to be applied; the questions asked in outcomes measurement; and, the continuum of effects included in the measurements.

REFERENCES

Agency for Healthcare Research and Quality. (1997). *CONQUEST*. Retrieved July 27, 2002, from http://www.ahcpr.gov/qual/conquest/conqovr1.htm
Agency for Healthcare Research and Quality. Outcomes Research. Fact Sheet. AHRQ Publication No. 00-P011, March 2000. Agency for Healthcare Research and Quality, Rockville, MD. http://www.ahrq.gov/clinic/outfact.htm
Australia Institute of Health and Welfare (2000). *Australia's Health 2000*. Canberra: Author.
Australia Institute of Health and Welfare and Commonwealth Department of Health and Family Services. (1997). *First report on national health priority areas 1996*. (AIHW Cat. No. PHE). Canberra: Authors.
Clancy, C. M., & Eisenberg, J. M. (1998). Health care policy–outcomes research: Measuring the end results of health care. *Science, 282*(5387), 245-246.
Cochrane Collaboration. (2002, July 24, 2002). *Cochrane Collaboration*. Retrieved July 27, 2002, from http://www.cochrane.org/
Donabedian, A. (1981). Criteria, norms, and standards of quality–what do they mean. *American Journal of Public Health, 71*(4), 409-412.
Government Performance and Results Act of 1993, Pub. L. No. 103-62; §1115, 107 Stat. 285. (1993).
Hurst, J., & Jee-Hughes, M. (2001, January 29). *Performance measurement and performance management in OECD health systems*. Organisation for Economic Co-operation and Development.
International City/County Management Association. (2002). *ICMA Center for Performance Measurement*. Retrieved July 26, 2002, http://icma.org/go.cfm? cid=1&gid=3&sid=101

Jee-Hughes, M., & Or, Z. (1999, January 21). *Health outcomes in OECD countries: A framework of health indicators for outcome-oriented policymaking.* Organisation for Economic Co-operation and Development.

Maloney, K., & Chaiken, B. P. (1999). An Overview of Outcomes Research and Measurement. In Coughlin, K. M. (2000). *2001 Medical outcomes and guidelines sourcebook.* New York: Faulkner & Gray.

Martin, L., & Kettner, P. (1996). *Measuring the performance of human service programs.* Thousand Oaks: Sage Publications.

Morley, E., Bryant, S., & Hatry, H. (2001). *Comparative performance measurement.* Washington, D.C.: The Urban Institute Press.

Mrazek, P., & Haggerty, R. J. (Eds.). (1994). *Reducing risks for mental disorders: Frontiers for preventive intervention research.* Washington, D.C.: National Academy Press.

Mullen, E. J. (2002a). *Evidence-based knowledge: Designs for enhancing practitioner use of research findings.* Paper presented at the 4th International Conference on Evaluation for Practice, University of Tampere, Tampere, Finland.

Mullen, E. J. (2002b). *Evidence-based social work–theory and practice: Historical and reflective perspective.* Paper presented at the 4th International Conference on Evaluation for Practice, University of Tampere, Tampere, Finland.

Mullen, E. J., & Bacon, W. F. (2002). Practitioner adoption and implementation of evidence-based effective treatments and issues of quality control. In A. Rosen & E. K. Proctor (Eds.), *Developing practice guidelines for social work interventions: Issues, methods, and a research agenda.* New York: Columbia University Press.

Mullen, E. J., Dumpson, J. R., & Associates (1972). *Evaluation of social intervention.* San Francisco: Jossey-Bass Publishers.

Mullen, E. J., & Magnabosco, J., (Eds.). (1997). *Outcomes measurement in the human services.* Washington, DC: National Association of Social Workers Press.

Murphy, L. L., Plake, B. S., Impara, J. C., Spies, R. A., & Buros Institute of Mental Measures (Eds.). (2002). *Tests in Print VI.* Lincoln, NE: Buros Institute of Mental Measurements, University of Nebraska-Lincoln: Distributed by the University of Nebraska Press.

Statistics Canada & Canadian Institute for Health Information (2001). *Health indicators April 2001.* Source: Statistics Canada's Internet Site, http://www.statcan.ca/english/freepub/82-221-XIE/00401/toc.htm, May 31, 2001.

United Kingdom Cabinet Report (2000). *Getting it together: A guide to public schemes and the delivery of public services.*

United Kingdom Clearing House on Health Outcomes. (March 1997). *Definitions of Outcomes.* Retrieved July 26, 2002, http://www.leeds.ac.uk/nuffield/infoservices/UKCH/define.html.

United Kingdom Office of the Deputy Prime Minister. (2002, July 23, 2002). *DTLR Best Value Site.* Retrieved July 26, 2002, from http://www.local-regions.odpm.gov.uk/bestvalue/bvindex.htm

United Kingdom National Health Service. (2000). *The NHS Plan.* Retrieved July 26, 2002, from http://www.nhs.uk/nationalplan/nhsplan.htm

United Nations Development Programme. (2000). *Human Development Report 2000.* New York & Oxford: Oxford University Press.

World Health Organization (2000). *The World Health Report 2000, Health Systems: Improving Performance.* Geneva: Author.

COMMUNITY AS A SOCIAL WORK ORIENTATION

Community Based Rural Health Care in India: Potential for Social Work Contribution

Sukla Deb Kanango

SUMMARY. India is a large country, geographically as well as populationwise. The majority of its population lives in rural areas, i.e., villages. Again, most of the villages are in remote areas. The State has been making sincere efforts to make the basic social services accessible to all in the rural area. Health being one of the vital services, it has been a challenging task before the State to extend it to the remote rural areas, many of which are not yet connected by motorable roads. As a result of various experiments carried out over the last five decades, the State has developed a fairly well-designed primary health care service, and it is in operation in rural areas. However, there appears to be a striking gap between the delivery

Sukla Deb Kanango, PhD, is Professor, Department of Social Work, Visva-Bharati, India (E-mail: jaharedeb@hotmail.com).

[Haworth co-indexing entry note]: "Community Based Rural Health Care in India: Potential for Social Work Contribution." Kanango, Sukla Deb. Co-published simultaneously in *Social Work in Mental Health* (The Haworth Social Work Practice Press, an imprint of The Haworth Press, Inc.) Vol. 2, No. 2/3, 2004, pp. 95-116; and: *Social Work Approaches in Health and Mental Health from Around the Globe* (ed: Metteri et al.) The Haworth Social Work Practice Press, an imprint of The Haworth Press, Inc., 2004, pp. 95-116. Single or multiple copies of this article are available for a fee from The Haworth Document Delivery Service [1-800-HAWORTH, 9:00 a.m. - 5:00 p.m. (EST). E-mail address: docdelivery@haworthpress.com].

Digital Object Identifier: 10.1300/J200v2n02_07

of health services in rural areas and utilization of the services by the people. Attempts have been made in this article to apprise the readers of the health service system in India, and it discusses the issue of health service delivery at the village level. The discussion is based on a small study carried out in a rural area in the State of West Bengal (India) where students of social work of the University to which the author belongs are placed for field work. Following the inputs received through supervision of the students' work, the study was initiated and conducted.

This article based on the study seeks to focus on peoples' perception of the health services as provided by the State in rural areas, which in turn gets reflected in the extent to which they utilize the services. Social workers being an integral part of the health set up, their role bears special significance. Discussion, therefore, centres on scope for social work intervention at the community level as well as in institutional level of the health service delivery system to make the services meaningful and effective in rural areas. In fact, it has to take the leadership role in reforming the service delivery system when required. *[Article copies available for a fee from The Haworth Document Delivery Service: 1-800-HAWORTH. E-mail address: <docdelivery@haworthpress.com> Website: <http://www.HaworthPress.com> © 2004 by The Haworth Press, Inc. All rights reserved.]*

KEYWORDS. Rural, State, Primary Health Centre, development block, health care service, West Bengal, service delivery, village, utilization, student, system, remote

INTRODUCTION

Investment in health is regarded as an important contributing factor to the development of a nation, not only in social terms but also in economic terms. A good health service is an asset of a society. For India, the health sector has been an important area in its total development endeavour. It has also been a serious concern for the State for the following reasons. India has a large population; compared to it the resources required to meet health needs are much less. The bulk of the population lives in rural areas and a large part of rural area in the country is remote and inaccessible in rainy seasons. Last but not least important are peoples' ignorance, apathy, and various myths and beliefs related to health practices. All these together have made the provision for health care service a challenging task for the State.

In addition, there is another major problem. As happens generally, all advanced and efficient systems of health services develop and get concentrated in big cities and towns. This has been the case in India also. As a result, the flow of people from the villages to towns and cities has become inevitable. This places unbearable pressure on the health services in urban areas. To reverse the process requires development of appropriate health care services in rural areas. Such services have to be of the kind that include preventive measures of sizable proportion along with curative services for ailments that do not require any complex system of treatment and can be safely treated in their place of origin. Keeping these two vital factors in view the State in India had established a well-designed network of primary health care services in rural areas. The present health service delivery system is now nearly more than three decades old. However, the service has been constantly subjected to intense public scrutiny and review, and reform of the delivery system is often demanded. The State attempts to respond to such situations but often its response falls far short of public expectations. A major issue in the health service delivery system in India lies here.

HEALTH CARE SYSTEM IN INDIA

In order to understand the health care system in India, it is useful to know the general administrative set-up in the country. Indian union is a federation of states (provinces). Various sectors' administration at the union and state level are regulated according to the jurisdiction laid down in the Indian Constitution. The sectors are grouped under three lists: (i) central list, which includes subjects exclusively administered by the union (central) government, e.g., defence, foreign policy, (ii) state list, which includes subjects that are exclusively under the domain of the states (provinces), e.g., law and order, (iii) concurrent list, which includes subjects which are within the purview of both union and state governments. Health is one such subject in the third list, so also education, social welfare, etc. In relation to the concurrent list, the union government provides the broad policy framework. It makes provision in the form of plan allocation, which is distributed among the states spread over the (five year) plan period. Each state, however, has the freedom to decide its own policy keeping in view its specific requirements within the national policy framework. Each state is also expected to mobilize its own resources to implement the programmes. Health being one of these, it may be helpful to know the health service set-up in India. For brevity and clarity, it is being presented in the form of a chart (see Chart I).

NATIONAL HEALTH POLICY

The National Health Policy (1983) evolved by the Ministry of Health and Family Welfare, Government of India, is being followed in designing health service development programmes at the state level.[1] The policy lays emphasis on the following aspects: prevention of ill-health, promotion of public health, curative, and rehabilitation services and primary health care services in remote areas.

In pursuit of these goals some of the noteworthy features of health programmes are:

a. supply of safe drinking water and basic sanitation using techniques that people can afford;
b. reduction of existing imbalance in health services by concentrating on the rural health infra-structure;
c. *concerted* action to combat widespread malnutrition; and
d. greater coordination of different systems of medicines.

Considering the major focus of this particular discussion, these areas bear special significance for rural health services in the country. Item (d) here needs little elaboration. India has a number of indigenous systems of medicine. Important among these are Ayurveda and Unani.[2] Ayurveda is called a science of life.[3] It teaches not only the art of living but also how to cure diseases totally and maintains the power to fight diseases. Apart from these, many other systems developed by various indigenous groups in different parts of the country are there. While they do not have a nomenclature by which they can be known, their utility has become all the more relevant today in the background of scarce resources and inaccessibility of modern systems of medicine *to* the majority of the people, particularly in rural areas.

Homeopathy is a comparatively later development in the country but nonetheless one of the most sought after systems of medicine for three main reasons–very nominal cost of treatment, easy accessibility, and *not* much paraphernalia of investigations needed for treatment.

In the State of West Bengal, which is the focus of the article, efforts are on to bring particularly Ayurveda and Homeopathy within the purview of the formal health care system in rural areas provided through the Primary Health Centres (PHC).

Another aspect that has a significant bearing on health and the health service delivery system is environment. It has become a matter of increasing concern, particularly for the health care system. Environmental hazards of urban areas are usually talked about, but environmental hazards of rural areas are no

CHART 1

HEALTH CARE SYSTEM IN INDIA*

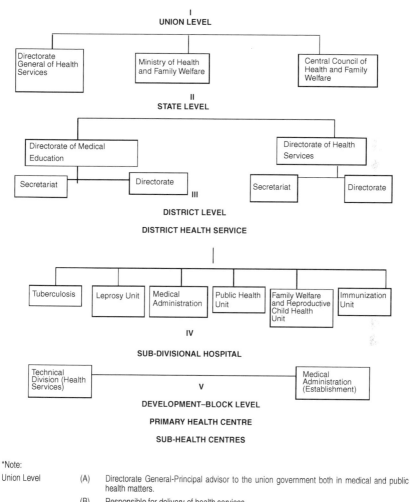

I
UNION LEVEL

| Directorate General of Health Services | Ministry of Health and Family Welfare | Central Council of Health and Family Welfare |

II
STATE LEVEL

Directorate of Medical Education
Directorate of Health Services

Secretariat   Directorate   III   Secretariat   Directorate

DISTRICT LEVEL

DISTRICT HEALTH SERVICE

Tuberculosis | Leprosy Unit | Medical Administration | Public Health Unit | Family Welfare and Reproductive Child Health Unit | Immunization Unit

IV

SUB-DIVISIONAL HOSPITAL

Technical Division (Health Services)   V   Medical Administration (Establishment)

DEVELOPMENT–BLOCK LEVEL

PRIMARY HEALTH CENTRE

SUB-HEALTH CENTRES

*Note:

Union Level	(A)	Directorate General-Principal advisor to the union government both in medical and public health matters.
	(B)	Responsible for delivery of health services.
	(C)	Considers recommendation of policies related to health services and distributes grants-in-aid to different states.
State Level	(a)	Responsible for policy decision.
	(b)	Responsible for policy implementation.
District, SubDivision Block Levels		Institutional set up responsible for health service delivery.

less disturbing. Lack of proper sanitation facilities, along with increasing use of chemicals in modern agricultural practice leading to pollution of *drinking water–the vital means of survival–*as well as the receding forest coverage and greeneries have made living in rural areas as threatening as other pollutants in urban areas, the difference *being* only of degree. This, therefore, is an important health service concern in the State. With the financial assistance from the World Health Organization, it is striving to improve its health service development programmes. Besides this, in collaboration with the UNICEF, a rural sanitation programme has been initiated to devise low-cost sanitary facilities that are/or can be within the means of rural people. Particularly the poor under this programme are helped with the subsidy provided by the government, and some NGOs have also taken the lead in this matter. However, voluntary participation of people in the programme is emphasized, and this, therefore, is a slow process.

HEALTH SERVICE SET-UP IN THE STATE OF WEST BENGAL

The health service set-up of the State of West Bengal is similar to the one described in the preceding chart. Promotion of health, prevention, and cure of disease form the three broad goals of health services in the State of West Bengal. Realization of the three goals becomes feasible when the service system is well managed. The state government lays special emphasis on the establishment of a dynamic health management system to make the health planning and health programme implementation meaningful. The approach adopted by the state is "bottom up," laying special emphasis on how the health-related situations can be taken care of at their places of origin (see Chart II).[4] The rationale behind this approach is to provide health facilities to treat common ailments at the village level itself. It also includes preventive measures such as mass immunization against childhood killer diseases and pre- and post-natal care of mothers. This is not only effective and meaningful but manageable, considering the limited resources (in material terms) available, while human and social support *from families and communities* are an added boon to this approach. Availability of such support is a remote possibility when treatment is carried out in a far-off health centre or hospital.

Administratively, there is a widespread network among health personnel at the grass roots level (see Chart III). This gets gradually consolidated and narrowed at the subsequent higher levels. Treatment of complex and complicated cases requiring specialized service then becomes the concern of the higher-level functional network.

CHART II

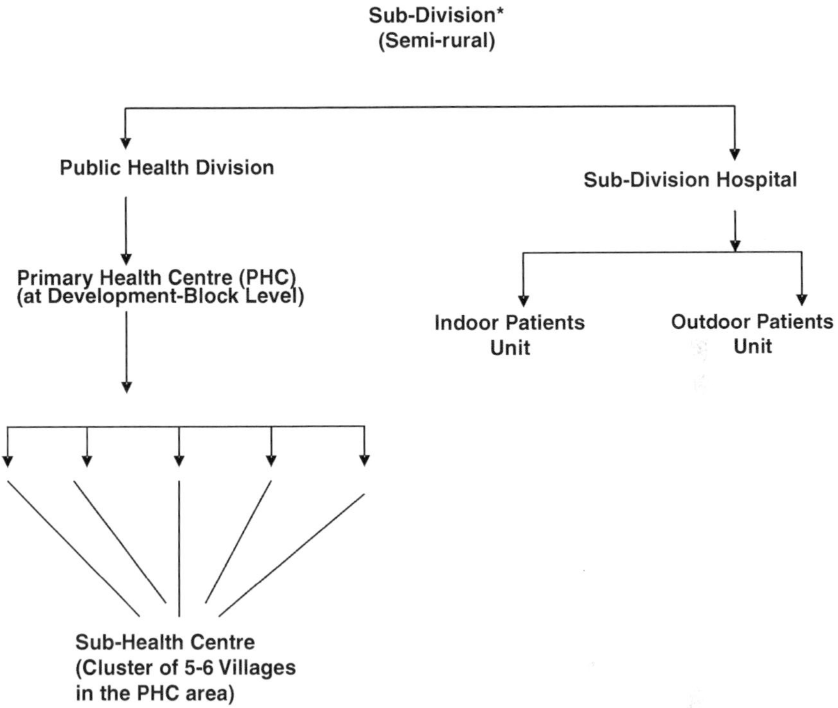

Sub-Division*
(Semi-rural)

```
                    ┌────────────────────────────────┐
                    ↓                                ↓
        Public Health Division
                    │                        Sub-Division Hospital
                    ↓                                │
  Primary Health Centre (PHC)              ┌─────────┴─────┐
  (at Development-Block Level)             ↓               ↓
                    │                 Indoor Patients  Outdoor Patients
                    │                      Unit             Unit
                    ↓
  ┌────┬────┬────┬────┬────┐
  ↓    ↓    ↓    ↓    ↓
   \    \   |   /    /
    \    \  |  /    /
     \    \ | /    /

        Sub-Health Centre
        (Cluster of 5-6 Villages
        in the PHC area)
```

*Level at which implementation of health programmes has direct bearing on people. As this goes down below primary health services, it is spread over to ensure that these reach remote areas.

However, as is the case, gaps between policy and programme implementation are universal phenomena and the State is no exception in this respect.

The subject matter of discussion in this article paper has a background. The article therefore, deals with this in the beginning, followed by the changes affecting health care, more particularly in rural areas of the country, their implications for social work practice and the position of social work leadership in the health care system.

Background

Social work intervention in the health care services of the State in rural areas *is* an inevitable part of field work assignments of the students of social

CHART III

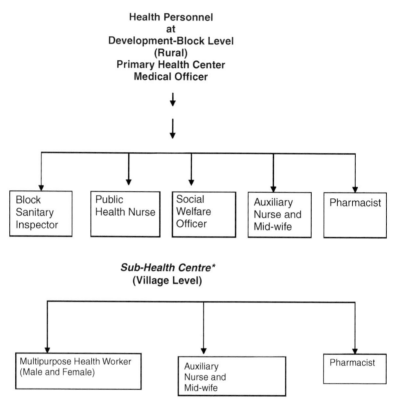

**Health Personnel
at
Development-Block Level
(Rural)
Primary Health Center
Medical Officer**

| Block Sanitary Inspector | Public Health Nurse | Social Welfare Officer | Auxiliary Nurse and Mid-wife | Pharmacist |

Sub-Health Centre*
(Village Level)

| Multipurpose Health Worker (Male and Female) | Auxiliary Nurse and Mid-wife | Pharmacist |

***There are three weekly clinics held at these levels—
(i) Tuberculosis, (ii) Leprosy, (iii) Mother and Child Health**

work of the University to which the author belongs. The field work programme is spread over 18-20 villages in the area and on an average, nearly 150 cases of health related difficulties are dealt with by the students in a year. While the programme's major focus is student learning, it has created a very good network among services rendered by the Primary Health Centres (PHC), health personnel in the field, other health agencies (private) in local area as well as social service division of major hospitals and teaching hospitals in cities and towns of the State. It built such confidence among the people that people often approach the faculty and students for referral to the bigger hospitals in the cities and towns.

At the village level, close collaboration with health staff facilitated effective teamwork in dissemination of health information, creation of awareness about health among the general public, and prevention and control of some prevalent common ailments and endemic diseases. This has been an important input in the service component at the village level, where social workers' major contribution lies and could be seen.

Brief mention of the following few cases (of hundreds) in which social workers' intervention helped mitigate the difficulties would explain the point.

A 35-year-old village priest suffering from congenital heart ailment was helped by the Social Worker to get the consultation of a leading cardiologist of a State Medical College and Hospital. He was advised to have surgery for replacement of a valve, to which the priest did not agree. He was apprehensive. He was counselled by the social worker all along this decision-making process. Ultimately, he was prescribed some medicines that he was required to take regularly. Being life saving drugs, these were available at a very nominal cost. His monthly expense in this regard was less than Rs.100.00 (a little more than U.S. $2.00). With this he carried on with his occupation quite normally.

The second case was of a child of 10 months suffering from a severe skin ailment. The family was extremely poor, and this was the first child of a young mother of 17 years. The social worker counselled her to hold patience and go for homeopathy treatment, which generally proved to be most effective as it killed the root cause of such diseases. Along with this she was advised to bathe the child with water in which margosa leaves, believed to contain antiseptic properties, were soaked well before bath. These had tremendous impact and the child was cured within a period of three months.

Third is the case of a village with a large number of tuberculosis patients. Social workers addressed the problem both at the individual level and at the community level. Most of the patients were drop-out cases. They were persuaded to resume treatment, while at the village level, a youth came forward to work in this area. He along with his peers took the initiative to uproot the disease from the village with the help of the social workers' guidance, advice, and referral. Already affected patients are cured and there is no case of tuberculosis in the village today.

In a country like India, which is always starved of resources, the above cases demonstrate the importance of *working at grass root levels in* (i) providing information and guidance, (ii) counselling at different stages of decision making, where required, and (iii) being there with the people and persons (families). In this way distressing problems could be solved in the most economical *way, avoiding* hazards of going for services from outside, *minimizing* expenses on treatment and preventing undue delay in commencement of treatment.

Such instances and many others proved the point that the holistic approach and aim at prevention of diseases are possible if social work takes the leadership or is given the leadership in the area. Prevention is such a vital approach for this country that it holds the possibility of taking care of health problems of millions of Indian people. Policywise, thrust has been shifting towards this area gradually. This has been the experience of student social workers working in the villages around the university. *However, policy* needs to be matched by the required practice in the field. Here is the vital area where the social worker's role and functions become significant.

HEALTH SERVICE DELIVERY AT VILLAGE LEVEL

Close examination of the system of delivery of health services, however, revealed certain important phenomena that needed serious consideration. It was, therefore, decided that systematic observation and collection of information pertaining to health service delivery from beneficiaries and health personnel would be necessary and useful. A small study was thus initiated. How the study was realized has been explained below.

As already mentioned, the study was conducted in the rural area where both undergraduate and post-graduate students of social work of the University to which the author belongs were placed for field work. One of the learning requirements in the courses was to learn the method of intervention by working with individuals and families. Invariably, while working with these people, the students were exposed to the problems of health and issues related to health services. Through supervisory conferences and, when need arose, through directly overseeing the student's work with individuals and families in the villages, some important issues came to light. Broadly, the issues were: In spite of well-designed primary health care set up in rural areas, people were having difficulties in getting proper services; tribal communities and people from poorer sections of the society were not much inclined towards the public health services; and lastly, the seemingly wide gap in the health personnel's response to communities' health service need.

As the study was conceived at a small scale it did not require any additional financial involvement. It could be managed within the regular schedule of work by investing some additional time to the task. Apart from three student social workers, one of the former post-graduate students (social work) of the University volunteered to be involved in the study. He had experience of working extensively in the area of community health as well as in a hospital setting at the sub-divisional level. Familiarity with the area and the people facilitated collection of relevant information without much time loss. Checking and re-checking of data were also quite easy.

SCOPE AND METHODOLOGY OF THE STUDY

On the basis of the observations made above it was decided to probe the following areas in the study:

i. Peoples' perception of the service they receive from the PHC *as regards its adequacy, inadequacy,* and quality of service;
ii. *Effective* working hours of the PHC, health personnel involved in delivery of services in the daily clinics and types of ailments with which patients attend the clinics;
iii. Health personnel, particularly the ones below the medical officer and the ones responsible for outreach programme in the villages, and their feelings about the health care set-up and the jobs that they have to perform;
iv. Sensitivity and concern of villagers about different health issues and the health services delivery system, if any, and their expectations;

The study was not of the conventional type. Methodology was the following:

a. Observation of working of the outdoor clinics (daily) of one *Primary Health Centre* over a period of a month with a gap of a day or two in between.
b. Observation of the special clinics like Mother and Child Health (MCH), Tuberculosis and Leprosy conducted by the *Primary Health Centre.*
c. Talk with the patients, using an interview guide, after they attended the clinics.
d. Talk with the health personnel of the *Primary Health Centre,* both at the clinics as well as in the field (using an interview guide).
e. Visit to five villages (randomly selected from among the villages in the operational area of the Primary Health Centre) and talk with groups of villagers on health issues and services rendered by the *Primary Health Centre.*

CATEGORIES OF PERSONS INVOLVED IN THE DISCUSSION WITH THE STUDENT SOCIAL WORKERS

a. Patients attending the daily clinics–patients were randomly picked out and included women, children (adolescent girls and boys), adult men, and old people, both male and female. Over the period of one month nearly 150 patients were talked to after they attended the clinics.

b. Health personnel–Auxiliary Nurse and Midwife (ANMs), Pharmacist and Health Assistants (Male and Female).
c. Villagers–five groups in five villages covered by different Subsidiary Health Centers (SHC). The modus operandi was that social workers started talking to two three persons whomever she/he came across and by the time the discussion set in motion many more people would join the discussion, first out of curiosity and then actively *through participation*. It, therefore, used to be a conglomeration of young and old but women were generally absent, in keeping with the village custom, where they were not expected or welcomed to enter into such deliberation along with their male counterparts. This aspect was therefore, taken care of by talking to women attending daily clinics at the *Primary Health Centre.*

WHAT THE STUDY REVEALED

Nature of treatment provided:

Irrespective of age and sex, patients came to the PHC with the following broad categories of ailments–fever, cold, cough; respiratory ailments; and diarrhoea and dermatological problems. On an average 50-60 patients daily came to the out-patient department. The working hours were from 9 a.m. to 12 noon and the doctor attended the clinics only on three days–from Monday to Wednesday and for three hours (daily) only. During the remaining three days of *the week,* clinics *were* conducted by the Auxiliary Nurse cum-Midwife themselves.

Discussion with the patients revealed that the PHC could provide only limited types and amounts of medicines, which was corroborated by the ANMs who mentioned that only 20 per cent of the required medicines were supplied by the PHC as that was what they were receiving from the government. Patients, therefore, were at the mercy of the drugstore and pharmacists. Most of the patients attending the clinics found this beyond their capacity to meet the cost of medicine. *To meet this demand, they resort to* borrowing or distress selling of their products such as cattle, harvest, and in some *instances,* even their land *provided they have some*.

Attempt was made to raise the issue of doctor not attending the clinics all six days in a week and if the people of the area intended doing anything about it. While the patients as well as the villagers (who participated in group discussion) appeared concerned about it, *they* expressed their helplessness as their appeal to the higher authority remained unanswered–'just ignored.' The *specious* ground on which the doctor declined to attend the clinics daily was that he was on contract and the contract amount was meager (only *Rs.6000.00 per* *month, U.S. $120.00 approximately*) which did not meet his bare requirements. While the regular employed medical officer of *the* government received four to five times more salary, the contract doctor could not be expected to render full, wholehearted service. The villagers seemed to get stuck at this argument and considered the doctor was justified in his action. What about themselves? Nothing much they could do about it, and it was left to their 'fate.'

RECEPTION OF PATIENTS

As far as reception of the patients *was concerned, they were subjected to* very abrasive and curt response if the patients were a little late in responding or unable to articulate their requirements. *These were generally the patients belonging to a tribal community and poorer and lower castes.* They also dropped-out of the treatment, mainly due to their economic hardships. *As was observed by Dr. D. Banerjee (2000), "Many of them reach a stage when they simply cannot afford to be ill, so they somehow drag on till it leads to serious . . ."* [5]

Therefore, *they were* not in a position to complete the full course of treatment. *No doubt, superstitions, ignorance, and impatience do play a significant part in this.* Especially when they did so and they were received with harsh verbiage from the health personnel. This further made them apprehensive and led to avoidance of the health centre as far as possible. If denied medicines, *in spite of these being there in the stock*, these patients could not *confront the health personnel for their reluctance to provide them with the service they were entitled to. They considered the situation as helpless, meaning thereby that they did not have the resources to change it.* This was the observation of the students also.

SERVICE GAPS

Service gaps in a number of situations were observed and reported by the health personnel themselves. For example, old people were seen to attend the clinics with cardiac problems when measurement of blood pressure was a requirement. If the doctor remained absent, the patients had to go without it. The instrument remained with the doctor. That means, if a patient came on a Thursday he had to wait till the next Monday for the doctor. The ANMs could easily do the job and advise the patients if the condition was not that serious. They were trained to *use the instrument* and *were* familiar with the general medicines prescribed for it. When confronted, *they would justify their action on the plea that they were not authorized by the doctor.* Unless this was brought to the notice of the doctor this would never get done. *If the pharmacist (who was in charge of the medicine store) also remained absent, the patients had to go without medicine.*

REFERRAL OF PATIENTS

Referral work was also seen to be greatly hampered as the doctor was not available most of the time and patients would not be entertained so easily, if the case was complicated, at the next higher institution, *viz.,* a sub-divisional hospital or a district-hospital. Most important, patients often would not know which specialized service section they should approach. *A social worker's presence here also would not help as only the doctor was authorized to make the referral.*

PATIENTS' OVERALL PERCEPTION AND SOCIAL WORKERS' OBSERVATION

Overall, the patients attending the PHC appeared to have had a feeling of inadequacy of services in general. However, their attitude towards the services was that at least they were getting some services closer home, they did not have to travel *miles to reach* a health facility which was the case earlier. It was also the observation of the social workers that the outreach programme of health was what people needed most in rural areas. The service delivery was designed in conformity with the 'bottom up' approach and people were aware that such a service existed. The need was how to make it meaningful, i.e., *to make the system* really work. Facilitating interpersonal communication among the health team was what was required most. On the other hand, it was essential that the patients who represented the community around the PHC did not remain only passive recipients of services but became active partners not only in utilizing the services but also in assisting the health teams in delivering their services in the right manner. Transparency in administration and service delivery would be possible when people exercised their right to know and at the same time, extended their judicious support to the health personnel. Social workers have a major role in sensitizing and organizing people to that effect. However, discrimination has to be made between becoming threatening and really well-meaning in realizing the rightful claims, what is called *'peoples' entitlement.* Social workers have to remain alert in this regard.

HEALTH PERSONNEL'S PERCEPTION

Within the physical set-up of health centres, health personnel were seen to be well accustomed to their routine functions and the patients also did not expect anything much beyond that from them. Health personnel's observation about the patients was that they lacked basic knowledge of maintaining good health and when ill, would not approach a health centre unless illness turned serious. However, the present approach of organizing outreach clinics was taking care of the following aspects quite *effectively*.

A Primary Health Centre area had been divided into zones and one Subsidiary Health Centre (SHC) had been established in each zone. Apart from this, the Health Assistants (both male and female), *also known as multi-purpose health workers*, conducted visits to the villages and administered iron tablets and vitamin A oil to the expectant mothers. Besides these, they advised the expectant mothers on pre-natal care. This, according to the health personnel, reduced the attendance of such women at the PHC and its clinics. Because of this reaching out, patients suffering from other simple ailments also got attended and hence the need to visit the PHC *became* less. However, a gap did exist here also. *People could get the service only if they approached the Health Assistant's*, and this often *did* not happen in many cases because people failed to approach them either due to negligence or lack of awareness. The health assistants' plea was that they could not attend to each and every person unless the individual approached them, which was justified to some extent. But it depended on the personality and approach of health personnel to make their presence felt so that the contact and communication between them and the people could take place easily.

An important area where, to a reasonable extent, integration of services had taken place, was the area of child health programmes. The Integrated Child Development Services Scheme, *operational* in the entire country and delivered at village levels, had health service and health education as integral components of its package of services.[6] The health personnel of the local area *Primary Health Centres were* responsible for providing these services. Because of the base being available at village level, *meeting of the two health* personnel and the children and pregnant and lactating *mothers* had become comparatively easy and quite effective. This *was* also an area which has succeeded in creating mass awareness to a considerable extent. This area focused on prevention whose impact *would* slowly become evident. In this particular area of study no systematic research *had* yet been conducted *but it is urgently needed*.

The two other specialized services rendered through the Primary Health Centres *were* Leprosy and Tuberculosis control and eradication. While the former, according to the health personnel, *had* become quite effective, the latter *was* suffering from many situational complications and drawbacks. *"Unconscious or conscious denial of the truth regarding the seriousness of the disease is a factor that leads to its neglect"*[7] *(Banerjee, 1968). This apart in poverty stricken families, patients, male or female, were busy earning their livelihood. "Going to a clinic for a check-up means losing several hours in queues and medical examinations and consequently the day's wage. They prefer postponement of diagnosis to immediate starvation."*[8] *The drawback in the programme was that all diagnostic tools were not available under one roof. For X-Ray, sputum and blood tests, patients had to travel to a government hospital, which was generally far off from most of the villages. It was only when diagnosed that medicines were supplied through clinics in the Primary Health Centres.*

The National Leprosy Elimination Programme had got a well-built set-up of reaching out to the patients.[9] The invention of Multi-Drug Therapy (MDT) *had* reduced the period of treatment substantially and the supply of this costly medicine was quite steady because of support from international organizations. Besides, the health personnel *were* required to administer the medicines directly to the patients in the out-patient clinics. Wherever feasible, voluntary social service organizations involved in the area of Leprosy control networking with them *was* an agreed policy of the State. This, therefore, *took* care of coverage to a considerable extent, areawise as well as populationwise.

Comparatively, tuberculosis control and eradication *had* been a difficult task. A host of factors, *apart from what has been mentioned previously*, contribute to this difficulty. Poverty coupled with complications arising out of Tuberculosis affected patients contracting Leprosy also *made* treatment very demanding. More so for patients because it *was* a long-term treatment and it required more resources, which a majority of the patients *did* not have. Mere supply of medicine free of cost *could not* ensure cure in these areas. Therefore, this area *had* remained an equally challenging one ever since the beginning of the programme. Patients' drop-out rate *was* very high in this case. It *was* draining of energy, effort, as well as all other resources. But all the same this *could* not be left out.

VILLAGERS' PERCEPTION OF HEALTH SERVICES

As mentioned already, five groups of villagers were met by the social workers in five different SHC zones. It needed some amount of prodding to make them sit down to discuss the health issues and health service delivery. It appeared that the villagers, in general, did not give much thought to the issues till these were brought to their attention by the social workers. The general comment about the PHC was that it should ensure the presence of a doctor on all days of a week and medicines should be supplied free of charge. They were not much bothered about the visits of the health personnel to the villages. The attitude was "if they come, well and good." Nothing much they thought about the advantage of such outreach work. Women's health was an important issue but for women remaining conspicuous by their absence, not much discussion could be pursued in this regard.

Student social workers' work with women and visit of the study team social workers to the homes of different women, however, brought the following issues to the fore. Most of these *were* common phenomena in developing countries such as India. Many of the difficulties of women lie with their inability to share their problems with their husbands and other elders in the family because of their inhibition. This *was* related mainly to *gynaecological* matters. Besides, they *were* unaware that for many such problems there *were* quite simple remedies available *in the Primary Health Centres*, and with proper knowledge, many complications in the area also *could* be prevented. Second, for the vast majority of women there *were* no proper toilet facilities available in their residences. As a result they either *had* to excuse themselves in the early morning or in the dark of night for the sake of privacy. This obviously *was* a health hazard that women in the villages suffered from. Third, it *had* been the observation of the students as well as study *team that the health needs of most of the women in villages were the last priority. Although the social system was responsible for this, women themselves were also responsible for their fate.* Women *considered* it as their responsibility to take care of others in the family first and then their own requirements. While menfolk *were* mindful of their needs, women *postponed* treatment till the last moment when it *went* beyond control. *For the menfolk, the only time they appeared concerned about women's health was when she was to deliver a child. They were least concerned if the period before and after the delivery went without complications.* The groups of people who met in the villages expressed the view that if the SHCs had facilities of maternity wards it would have been really helpful to them.

Environmental hazards to women's health *were* many in rural areas. Day after day they *were* carrying loads of firewood and travelling miles together for collecting the same. Sometimes women carried their infants or small children along with them when they *went* out to collect the firewood. Hence it *was* a back-breaking job for them. Besides, the environment within home *was* also not without hazards. Cooking being done on firewood, and lighting using kerosene oil, *made* them spend a large part of their time in the smoke that emanated from these. This put severe strain on their eyes apart from the fact that they inhaled the smoke. Those women who *worked* in the farm and field *were* exposed to the chemical hazards of modern agricultural practices but they *had* no other alternative before them.

Hence, women's health *was* an area about which the village community in general *was* not much concerned, but it demanded the serious attention of the policy makers and planners in health to help remove the hazards related to health of women in rural areas.

In summing up, it may be said that the health service delivery system (formal) at the community level indicated the following broad reasons for under-utilization and non-utilization of services by the people:

a. non-availability of qualified medical practitioners at the health centres as and when people need their service;
b. supply of nominal amount of medicine free of charge, otherwise most of the drugs are to be purchased from the open market;
c. service gap;
d. poor reception

At the same time it must also be mentioned that a comparatively lesser number of people visit the PHC as a quite systematic outreach programme has been developed at the village level.

As already mentioned, the author, being acquainted with the people and culture of the area through *her* interaction with them, is familiar with certain health practices and peoples' attitudes towards health services. Apart from what has been explained previously, following are some of the observations, which may not be out of place to mention here.

Poverty apart, villagers mostly do not follow the full course of treatment prescribed and often expect immediate results. This obviously cannot be guaranteed by anybody. Hence very soon they lose confidence in the treatment provided by the Primary Health Centre and dub it as 'useless.' On the other hand, since the illness persists they fall back on folk remedy. Some times folk remedies do produce good results, but in many cases they complicate the situations. It takes lot of effort and time to reason with them. It is not only that large numbers of manpower are required to deal with this dimension of health practices in the villages, it is also beyond the means of the State to provide such types of quality service should have intensive counselling component. *The* medical social workers can provide this but it is a highly time consuming work *and costly affair*. It also needs follow-up for a long period.

The Primary Health Service network is now quite widespread. Even then one Primary Health Centre serving a cluster of twenty to twenty-five villages is not equally accessible to all. A sizeable number of villages are connected by non-metalled and non-motorable road with the Primary Health Centre. This acts as a deterrent to going to the Centre. It is time consuming, laborious in that people have to walk a long distance in the absence of suitable transport facilities. These are situational limitations in the face of which both State and people are helpless.

While these are realities, some are within the power of the people to take care of. They need to change their outlook so far as the conditions are concerned. Since health is an important aspect of human existence, the distance of the Health Centre or *not following the full course of treatment on the pretext of its ineffectiveness cannot be a defence for not* going for treatment by qualified trained health personnel. Often health personnel, from Medical Officer to field staff (grass root level functionaries) are blamed. The major irritant to the doctors and other health personnel is complications of illness condition due to negligence, ignorance, superstitions, and delayed approach for services *by the villagers in general.* Under such circumstances health personnel can do precious little to cure the patients. On the one hand, the burden of large numbers of patients and on *the* other, scarce resources, *including manpower*, make the job of balancing the delivery system extremely difficult for them and they are often blamed for poor service delivery.

SOCIAL WORKERS' LEADERSHIP ROLE

Social work leadership would imply the initiative and concerted action that the social work profession had to take both in terms of formulating appropriate new policy or modifying the existing one as well as mobilizing the services of the medical profession wherever it was needed, in addition to providing counselling for prevention and amelioration of difficulties related to health. In preventive and promotive health work, social workers play the crucial role by initiating and establishing such services. In the context of the present discussion, this leadership would imply finding and realizing space within the existing public health service set-up to initiate the required change and bring improvement in extending the services to the people, helping them make use of it in an appropriate manner, and where needed, mobilization at the community level to bridge the service gap.

Although the facts revealed by the study here were more or less known, going for this at this stage helped in learning about peoples' perceptions of the contemporary scenario and *the kinds of benefits they accrue to the common people by the newly reorganized set-up.* This also reinforced the belief that social workers have a vital role to play in the area. It may be mentioned that the Social Welfare Officer (who is generally a trained social worker) of Development

Blocks plays a lead role in planning and organizing the community level services (on a mass scale) such as immunization, family planning, health camps, reproductive health programmes for women and adolescents, etc. However, the social workers being very negligible in number–there is only one Social Welfare Officer in the Development Block–the issues thrown up by the study can not be taken care of.

In the background of this study one can visualize the following areas in which social workers have to play a pivotal role:

Policy changes: Both minor and major policy changes are required in the delivery of health services. Service gaps provide the indicator at which these are to be directed. While government's approach is target oriented, mere targets do not generally make a quality impact on the services. What is needed is the clear focus, not only on the target population but also on the approach that would make the qualitative change. Often the target is unreachable and somehow the job is done. Instead, it is required to focus on manageability of the issues taken up. These would require working at major policy changes.

While working with the other members of the health team, often minor changes are to be made to plug the service gap. This, therefore, requires working with the member concern to facilitate the desired change in the policy, e.g., the case of measuring blood pressure as noted earlier.

Service utilization: The first requirement is providing information to people about the availability of service and the procedural requirements to be fulfilled to gain access to the service. Lack *of information is responsible for non-utilization.* Here, social workers only can take the lead. Information is power, and armed with information, the majority of the people can decide for themselves. There has been ample proof of it. When well informed, people can reach out for the service, and that is the real need in the approach by the health professionals.

Second, people suffer from a lot of apprehensions regarding the outcome of various types of treatment. This is also a vital area where people need to be informed about the pros and cons of treatment outcome so that they can make judicious decisions. *Also, they have to be sensitized about their responsibility, which they must fulfil, e.g., to follow the prescribed treatment fully.*

Third, for people in rural areas the mere establishment of a service is not enough. Even, being the single provider of health service, government health set-ups remain considerably unutilized by the people, reasons for which have become quite evident in this study (mainly irregular attendance of doctors and non-availability of most of the medicines). Hence, reaching out to people to some extent is essential, apart from supply of reasonable *health care support.* Cordiality in reception can make marked qualitative changes in the delivery of health services in rural areas.

Counselling and guidance form the vital components in utilizing services by the people, more particularly the marginalized and disadvantaged sections. These are to be provided by the social workers as the others in the health team have very little desire, acumen, and time to do so.

Protection of Patients' Rights: The first area of concern here is the patient's right to information when a specific course of treatment is prescribed. Very *rarely* is this right of the patients recognized by the medical profession. Here the social worker has to intervene and ensure that patients make a decision after being informed well about the line of treatment and its prognosis.

Although, at the community level in the rural areas, violation of peoples' rights as consumers of services may not be very apparent, advocacy to ensure peoples' right to get the services is an important task of social work professionals *working in a health related field.*

Prevention

Health education and awareness, whose advantages need reinforcement through social workers' intervention, is vital. This is particularly essential for rural areas as education and awareness can prevent many of the maladies and make 'management of health' manageable. Social workers have a significant role to play in this respect. This is well recognized, but then social workers have to create space for themselves as State support (financial) is most unlikely. The State is engaged in the biggest struggle of providing primary health care services, although preventive care is valued. For a country such as India, engagement of social workers by the State in each Sub-Health Centre is impossible, but that is what is desirable and required.

CONCLUSION

Health care service is one of the vital services provided by the State, which should take care of the entire population. It should be relevant to all. Considering the large size of population and volume of services required, it is a challenging task for the State as well as for the health professionals responsible for administering the services. The majority of the people of the country being based in a rural area, it has been a constant exercise by the State *as to how* to make the services accessible and meaningful to the people. Various models have been tried over the period. Some have shown positive results but these have been gradual and comparatively slow. The bulk of the people remain indifferent towards states' health services. *While private health services do serve the people better, only a few can afford it. Also, these are mostly not available in rural area.* Under the circumstances it is imperative that the public health services have to be made to work. This is possible only when people become partners in the delivery of services. This, in other words, means people need to be organized around the issue. This can be attempted only *with* the initiative of social work professionals coupled with *state's* support to let people become partners and participate. *Only then will the revamping of health services in rural areas be possible.*

REFERENCES

1. Government of India, Ministry of Health and Family Welfare, *Statement on National Health Policy*, New Delhi, 1983.

2. Bijlani, Ramesh: *Yoga and Health*, Health for the Millions, May-June 1999 Vol. 25, No. p. 3, pp. 12-13.

3. Chandra, Shailaja: *Can Public Health and Traditional Medicine Meet or Mix?*, Health for the Millions, September-October, 2000, p. 16.

4. Health Service Set up in the State of West Bengal: Document for internal circulation in the S. D. Hospital–source, Superintendent, S. D. Hospital, Bolpur, West Bengal.

5. Banerjee, D: *Decaying health services and the increasing suffering of the voiceless* Health for the Millions, Jan.-Feb., 2000, Vol. 26, No. p. 1, p. 34.

6. Relief and Welfare Department, Government of West Bengal: *Handbook on Integrated Child Development Services Scheme in West Bengal* (year not mentioned), pp. 19-23.

7. Banerjee, G. R.: *The Tuberculosis Patient*, Tata Institute of Social Sciences, Bombay, 1968, p. 18.

8. *Handbook on Eradication of Leprosy*, WHO Standard Multi-Drug Therapy (M.D.T) in Bengali, WHO, New Delhi, India (year not mentioned).

Tackling Problem Drug Use:
A New Conceptual Framework

Julian Buchanan

SUMMARY. Successful 'recovery' from long-term problem drug use has depended largely upon understanding and tackling the physiological and psychological nature of drug dependence; however, drawing upon research and practice in Liverpool, England, the author questions whether this discourse is sufficient given the changing nature, context and attitudes towards drug consumption in the twenty-first century. This article emphasises the importance of incorporating structural and social factors. Drawing upon qualitative data from three separate studies, the author illustrates how stigmatisation, marginalisation, and social exclusion are significant debilitating components that have tended to be overlooked. This paper contributes new insights into the damaging impact of political rhetoric and structural discrimination that has placed many long-term drug users vulnerable to relapse. In response to these findings the author offers a new conceptual framework for practice that incorporates and pro-

---

Julian Buchanan, Cert PA, DipSW, MA, is Senior Lecturer/Researcher in Social Welfare and Community Justice, University of Wales, Wrecsam, Wales, LL11 2AW (E-mail: julian.buchanan@ntlworld.com).

The author is indebted to Lee Young whose many hours of discussion and rigorous analysis helped to shape and develop the thinking behind this paper, and to colleagues at University of Wales, Wrecsam for their help and advice.

[Haworth co-indexing entry note]: "Tackling Problem Drug Use: A New Conceptual Framework." Buchanan, Julian. Co-published simultaneously in *Social Work in Mental Health* (The Haworth Social Work Practice Press, an imprint of The Haworth Press, Inc.) Vol. 2, No. 2/3, 2004, pp. 117-138; and: *Social Work Approaches in Health and Mental Health from Around the Globe* (ed: Metteri et al.) The Haworth Social Work Practice Press, an imprint of The Haworth Press, Inc., 2004, pp. 117-138. Single or multiple copies of this article are available for a fee from The Haworth Document Delivery Service [1-800-HAWORTH, 9:00 a.m. - 5:00 p.m. (EST). E-mail address: docdelivery@haworthpress.com].

motes an understanding of the social nature and context of long-term drug dependence. *[Article copies available for a fee from The Haworth Document Delivery Service: 1-800-HAWORTH. E-mail address: <docdelivery@haworthpress.com> Website: <http://www.HaworthPress.com> © 2004 by The Haworth Press, Inc. All rights reserved.]*

KEYWORDS. Drugs, social exclusion, substance misuse, drug abuse, addiction, discrimination, social work

INTRODUCTION

Based on twenty years research and practice with dependent drug users in Liverpool, England the author argues that a new paradigm is required to inform social welfare intervention with long-term dependent drug users. Existing theoretical perspectives promoted in the 1960s and 1970s such as the 12-step programme, cycle of change, Methadone Maintenance Therapy, inpatient detoxification, and therapeutic communities all have considerable merit. They continue to be used with varying degrees of success, but they remain heavily based upon physiological and psychological perspectives with the emphasis upon motivation, commitment and tackling physical dependency. This paper draws upon three separate qualitative research studies in Liverpool, that involved semi-structured interviews with 200 known problem drug users. The studies recognised the importance of user led research and for policy makers to listen to the messages from the users' themselves. These studies sought to ascertain the views, suggestions and experiences of drug users in respect of what was helping or hindering them from giving up a drug dominated lifestyle. The findings suggest that the significant social and cultural changes in the late 20th century have diluted the impact and effectiveness of traditional approaches to assist long term dependent drug users. Drawing upon the messages from the drugs users themselves, this article will highlight the debilitating nature of marginalisation and social exclusion that many long term problem drug users have experienced. It concludes by suggesting a new social model to understand and conceptualise the process of recovery from drug dependence, one that incorporates social reintegration, anti-discrimination and traditional social work values.

CHANGING NATURE AND CONTEXT

In the 1960s and 1970s, drug use in the UK was largely isolated and confined to a relatively small section of society that tended to use drugs as a symbol of protest and rebellion (Royal College of Psychiatrists 2001). At the same time many saw illicit drug use as a potentially dangerous and deviant activity, which was to be avoided. However, the past 30 years have seen rapid social change, nationally and globally. In many countries taking illegal drugs is now regarded as one of many adolescent experiences. In the UK, 49 per cent of young people aged 16 to 29 admit to taking a prohibited drug (Ramsay & Partridge 1999 p. viii). A longitudinal study involving a sample of over 500 teenagers from schools in North West England identified that, by the time they had reached the age of 18 years old, over 64% had tried an illegal drug (Parker et al. 1998 p. 85). Illegal drugs are now easily accessible in virtually any part of the UK through carefully developed networks, greatly assisted by the widespread use and availability of mobile phones (May et al., 2000). Knowledge and understanding of the true nature and risk of illegal drugs is improving, particularly in relation to cannabis. There is more of a willingness to speak openly, for example the Independent Inquiry by the UK Police Foundation stated:

> *But by any of the main criteria of harm–mortality, morbidity, toxicity, addictiveness, and relationships with crime–it [cannabis] is less harmful to the individual and society than any other of the major illicit drugs, or than alcohol and tobacco.* Police Foundation (2000 p. 7)

While recreational use of cannabis can, for some people, be relatively unproblematic, other drugs, such as heroin and crack cocaine, are more likely to lead to difficulties and dependence. What is interesting is that many young people are making well-informed risk assessments when deciding which drugs they use, with cannabis, poppers and amphetamine being the most popular (Measham et al. 2001). This awareness and distinction between different illegal substances doesn't appear to be acknowledged or recognised by a UK government rhetoric that prefers a 'blanket' approach: "*All drugs are harmful and enforcement against all illegal substances will continue*" (Her Majesty's Government 1998:3), though more recently some distinctions are beginning to emerge with the proposed reclassification of cannabis.

For many decades alcohol and tobacco have been the established and heavily promoted recreational drugs of choice, but as with many other 'pillars' of social life this dominant 'cultural choice' is being challenged. Some individuals and sections of society have already made informed choices to select different recreational drugs, albeit ones that are currently categorised as illegal. Indeed, uncertainty, choice, diversity, and risk taking have become key themes of postmodern life. In this context it becomes much easier to view taking illicit drugs as just another of many life choice options, all involving inherent risks and benefits. Regrettably, some of the most dangerous risks to taking illegal drugs are by-products of the illegal status of the drug, rather than the substance itself. It can be argued that many young people are choosing substances that are, if a clean legal supply could be obtained, far less damaging than the heavily promoted commercial substances, alcohol and tobacco.

While society and the nature and extent of drug taking have changed significantly over the past two decades, the approach to the problem of illicit drugs in the UK has not sufficiently adapted to take into account this changing social, political and economic environment. The UK government's 10-year drug strategy (Her Majesty's Government 1998) promotes the 'war on drugs' rhetoric and sets out to eradicate the so-called 'menace' and 'threat' of any substance that is not legal. This has led to a closer alliance between the UK and the U.S. In both countries, drug policy and drug treatment are locked into the criminal justice system resulting in escalating numbers of drug users held in overcrowded prisons. Both countries are experiencing a prison crisis with numbers escalating out of control. In 1990 the U.S. incarcerated 458 people per 100,000 residents; by the year 2000 it had risen to a staggering 699 people per 100,000. The rate of incarceration increased so much in the U.S. since they declared 'war on drugs' that apart from Russia, the U.S. now incarcerates more of their people than any other nation in the world (U.S. Department of Justice 2001). In 1990, the prison population in England and Wales was 46,504; by the year 2000 it had increased drastically to 65,993; 125 people per 100,000 residents. While significantly less than the U.S., the UK now has the second highest incarceration rate in the European Union (Hansard 1990, Walmsley 2000). A recent survey indicated that 51 per cent of males now on remand and 54 per cent of female remand reported a drug dependency problem (DoH 2001). The use of the criminal justice system and, ultimately, incarceration to tackle widespread illicit drug consumption in post modern society is increasingly under scrutiny and criticism from a wider audience. *The Lancet* commented:

> *Since the 1970s, the USA has spent billions in a largely futile effort to stem the influx of drugs, imprisoned hundreds of thousands of men and women, many with long sentences for minor offences, and poured billions into media and school-based education campaigns of questionable effectiveness.* (Lancet Editorial 2001)

As illicit drug use becomes a mainstream activity, drug policies that lean heavily upon the criminal justice system to wage war on drugs are creating a spiralling prison population and a growing concern regarding human rights violations, as Karim Murji explains:

> the view that the state has a paternalistic duty to stop people from harming themselves by taking drugs is contradictory and incoherent, since

there are other potentially harmful activities, for example, people engaging in dangerous sports, that are not treated in the same way. (Murji 1998 p. 56)

Illicit drug taking has become an accepted life choice, particularly amongst the under 40s, while at the same time, those in power (usually the over 40s) attempt to persuade society that all illegal drugs are dangerous and that people should unite to eradicate them. This promotes the illusion that such a goal is not only morally 'right,' but also achievable. The creation of this divisive 'moral high ground' of legal drug users (alcohol and tobacco) has serious implications and consequences for illegal drug users and drug workers who observe a growing chasm between the rhetoric concerning the risks and dangers of drugs, and the reality of their own personal experiences.

In recent years UK political parties have been competing with one another to be seen to be winning the political war on drugs by developing tougher and less tolerant policies (Buchanan & Young 1998), such as the recently introduced Drug Treatment and Testing Orders, and Abstention (*and drug testing*) Orders for offenders susceptible to taking illegal drugs. Inevitably, this not only results in harsher and less humane policies and practices, but also a hardening of attitudes towards those dependent on illegal drugs. In maintaining power and winning political popularity, governments' benefit by creating enemies that they then can be seen to be protecting their people from. Societies can then unite, waging war against 'suitable enemies' (Christie 1986), and drug users have become a convenient group to demonise (Van Ree 1997). Some of the harshest government policies towards drugs and drug users in recent years have been located in the United States and some of the Nordic countries. Within these countries some academics like Trebach (1987) in the United States, and Christie and Bruun (1985) in the Nordic countries have questioned the rationale and validity of such hostile and counterproductive policies. Their criticism of harsh drug policies that promote war against illegal drugs has, sadly, not always been welcomed or appreciated

In countries that wage war on the enemy of illegal drugs, those who are given the label 'druggie' or 'smackhead' find themselves not only socially marginalised and isolated, but subject to hostility and distrust. The war on drugs is a war on drug users, a civil war against an enemy within (Buchanan & Young 2000). Within this climate, attempts by recovering dependent drug users to find understanding, friendship, and other opportunities to socially reintegrate with the wider population tend to quickly fail. This reality and the impact of this experience need careful understanding if agencies, are to effectively assist dependent drug users on the road to recovery. The social dimension has been largely overlooked by 'treatment' agencies, which have concentrated upon tackling the physiological and psychological aspects of dependency, along with a growing emphasis (promoted by the involvement of correctional agencies), to protect society.

THE LIMITATIONS OF A PHYSIOLOGICAL APPROACH

Some physiologically dependent drug users are so intoxicated and out of control that it is difficult for them to make rational choices until they become drug free, a situation not uncommon with heavy long-term use of alcohol, heroin or benzodiazepines. However, some professionals wrongly perceive illegal drugs as inherently 'bad' to the extent that rational decision making is not possible until the person becomes drug free, and that illegal drugs are incompatible with a normal healthy life. Abstinence based workers see the removal of all illegal substances from the blood stream as the *only* viable option for recovery. Once 'addicts' are detoxed they gain the status of an 'ex-addict,' and this status can be regularly and randomly monitored by increasingly more sophisticated drug testing on blood, urine, saliva, hair, etc.

Abstentionists tend to regard clean legal substitute drugs as a poor alternative, because the person is still physically dependent, and concern is expressed because methadone is just as addictive as heroin itself (Robson 1999). While this is physiologically accurate, it is potentially misleading because it presents drug dependency within a medicalised conceptual framework that sees drug dependence as essentially a physical addiction. This has implications for policy and practice. For example, in Merseyside, England, so convinced by the need to set her son free from physical dependence upon the 'evils' of heroin, one parent literally chained her son to the banister rail so he was restricted and only able to wander between his bedroom and the bathroom. This continued for three weeks until he became physically drug free, and therefore an ex-addict. Other strategies to become drug free have included holidays abroad to physically withdraw, while others have sought imprisonment (though this can hardly be regarded as a drug free environment). To those who place heavy emphasis on the physiological nature of dependence, it comes as something of a shock (as many drug users have testified) to discover the cravings, the stomach cramps and sweats can all come flooding back once set free and back in the original environment where they are exposed to well-established psychological and social cues and triggers. It doesn't seem to matter how long the person was away from the environment, or how long they have been drug free. When the young man who was chained to the banister rail was released by his mother, he immediately returned to his heroin habit.

While the physiological aspect of problem drug use needs to be taken seriously, it is clearly just one component of drug dependence. It does not in itself provide an adequate understanding of dependence, and can lead to the exclusive promotion of abstinence-only programmes, suggesting that harm reduction merely condones or prolongs drug taking. However, many dependent drug users are able to live normal and healthy lives while maintained on legally prescribed substitute drugs (McDermott 2001), but sadly, access to clean legal drugs is severely limited, and many Health Authorities are unwilling to provide clean injectable drugs. The preoccupation with physical withdrawal can also lead to a failure to recognise other crucial aspects of dependence. Drucker highlights this point:

> *In an environment frightened with powerful moral and legal reactions to the use of drugs, the stigma attached to drugs may come to be a more important factor than the biology of addiction, the demonization of drugs and the criminalization of the drug user (i.e., the war on drugs) could be more damaging to the individual and society than drug use or addiction.* (Drucker 2000 p. 31)

THE NEED FOR A PSYCHOLOGICAL APPROACH

In response to the limitations of a physiological approach, psychologists have usefully identified and introduced various cognitive behavioural theories to the field of drug dependence, including social learning theory (Bandura 1977), cognitive therapy (Beck 1979), motivational interviewing (Miller & Rollnick 1991) and the cycle of change (Prochaska et al. 1992). These insights have enabled a more complete understanding of the nature of drug dependence beyond the limited understanding of physical addiction. This has provided new knowledge in understanding triggers, craving, relapse, the development of learnt (habitual) behaviour, and of particular importance, the assessment of motivation. Incorporating the psychological dimension has enabled more productive work to be carried out with a wider range of drug users, including those who are not necessarily wanting to become drug free, but seeking help to regain control over aspects of their life.

The integration of the physiological and the psychological dimensions of drug dependence largely informed the treatment of UK dependent drug users. Policy has also been influenced by a pragmatic strategy of 'harm reduction' promoted by the Government Advisory Committee in the late 1980s (Advisory Council on the Misuse of Drugs 1988). This strategy was based on the premise that HIV posed a greater threat than drug use itself; therefore, agencies had to be prepared to accept continued drug use in order to develop relationships with the drug using community and encourage safer practices to protect the spread of infection to the non drug using population. Controversially, this involved the supply of free clean needles/syringes, free condoms, and maintenance prescribing of substitute drugs. Some clinicians even prescribed amphetamine and heroin to dependent drug users, sometimes in injectable form (ampoules). Harm reduction was reluctantly embraced as agencies felt obliged by their responsibility to protect the non-drug using population from the risk of HIV/AIDS (Riley & O'Hare 2000). However, as the incidences of AIDS cases related to injecting drug use began to fall significantly in the mid 1990s across EU countries (European Monitoring Centre For Drugs And Drug Addiction 1999), interestingly, so has the prominence and practice of harm reduction. This is not surprising given that harm reduction has not been accepted by the United Nations Drug Abuse Control and Crime Prevention (UNDCCP). Hartnoll identifies the problem of harm reduction for some countries such as the United States government:

> *it lacks commitment to a drug free goal, accepts, or condones continued use of drugs, and implies a hidden agenda of decriminalisation or legalisation.* (Hartnoll 1998 p. 240)

UK practice with drug users has, then, been shaped by three separate frameworks of understanding: physiological dependence, psychological approaches, and the pragmatic philosophy of harm reduction. The promotion of harm reduction resulted in more accessible and appropriate 'user friendly' services for drug users, but the actual practice of harm reduction tended to be limited and often confined to narrow health interpretations. While the physiological approach tended to subscribe to pathological notions of dependence promoting ideas of the 'demon' drink or drug, the psychological approaches also run the risk of decontextualising dependent drug users, suggesting dependence can largely be controlled by internal adjustments in thinking, motivation or the development of cognitive behavioural techniques. All three frameworks offer an important contribution, but they each give limited attention to the social, political and economic context of drug taking in postmodern society. Many socially excluded dependent drug users in the UK struggle to break out of a drug centred existence, even when they become physically drug free and display an abundance of psychological insight and self-motivation. These drug users face a more difficult challenge of overcoming the many layers of discrimination and social exclusion, which have become a by-product of government rhetoric and policy on drugs.

GETTING TOUGH ON DRUG USE

In the mid-1990s the UK government abandoned the pragmatic 'British System,' which was largely based upon prescribing heroin and substitute drugs through treatment in the Health Service (South 1997), which had for so long been the backbone of UK practice, and shifted to the U.S. model with a focus upon compulsory treatment, and abstinence through the Criminal Justice System. Interestingly, government press releases began using dramatic language describing drugs as a scourge on communities, as the cause of most criminal offences, the cause of family breakdown, a social menace, and a threat to the fabric of society. Tony Blair, UK Prime Minister, called on the nation to *'break once and for all the vicious cycle of drugs and crime which wrecks lives and threatens communities'* (Her Majesty's Government 1998 p. 3). As the rhetoric gathers momentum, the focus of unease, the personification of the drug problem is clearly targeted at drug users and drug pushers. A press release from the UK Treasury Department announcing £300 million to fight drugs stated;:

> *hardly a family is unaffected by the evil of drugs . . . Drug-related crime blights our communities. It destroys families and young lives and fuels a wide range of criminal activity, including burglary and robbery. . . We won't tolerate the menace of drugs in our communities–it causes misery and costs lives. . . This new money will enable agencies to step up their fight against drugs and the crime it breeds. It will get drug dealers off our kids' backs and into prison and help safeguard our communities. (HM Treasury 2001)*

What is missing is an understanding that those who trade on drugs are in the majority of cases those who have also become dependent upon drugs. Most users tend to buy for or sell to friends at some point or other, despite the fact that the offence of supplying drugs carries a lengthy prison sentence. The distinction between user and pusher is not as clear as it is portrayed.

The War on Drugs rhetoric promoted by ex-Prime Minister Lady Thatcher, has served to demonise, isolate and discriminate against drug users. The institutionalised use of prejudice, power and propaganda to promote discriminatory thinking towards anyone using illegal substances is highly questionable. History tells us that other groups have endured similar experiences, such as black people, gay/lesbian people, travellers and women, and many continue to do so. Not before time, many of these discriminatory perspectives have been challenged (Thompson 2001), and the damaging and offensive stereotypes have been exposed, though further work is still needed.

Sadly, while progress is made to tackle discrimination to one group, new groups emerge, such as drug users, who are subject to *personal, cultural, and structural* (Thompson 2001) discrimination. Like many other discriminated groups, some drug users have internalised the negative and harsh stereotypes imposed upon them, leaving them with poor confidence, low self-esteem, low aspirations and little self-worth (Buchanan & Young 1996). Social work seeks to combat discrimination in all forms, but the experiences of drug users tend to go largely unnoticed and are rarely mentioned as a discriminated group.

DRUG USERS–A SCAPEGOAT?

Drawing upon three separate qualitative research studies (Goldson et al., 1995, Buchanan & Young 1996, Buchanan & Young 1998a) involving semi-structured interviews with 200 known problem drug users in Merseyside illustrates how the war on drugs has served to legitimise and reinforce structural discrimination against drug users. The three commissioned research studies involved listening to the views of problem drug users with a common shared aim to identify the barriers that hinder their capacity to regain control of their drug habit, and to listen to the suggestions from the drug users themselves about improvements in services to enable social reintegration. The first two studies led to the establishment of Day Centre provision (Bootle, Merseyside) and a Structured Day Programme (Liverpool, Merseyside). The third study involved action research: interviewing the drug users who attended the Structured Day Programme, listening and recording their experiences. The studies all placed importance upon listening to the drug users and sought through the research to give them a voice. Common themes emerged from the drug users interviewed in these three studies:

- Their social dislocation
- Their poor experiences of education and employment
- Their lack of realistic opportunities and hope
- Their isolation from a non-drug-using population
- A sense of stigma and low self-esteem

This article seeks to promote the voice of the drug users involved in the research. Allowing their messages concerning the impact that social exclusion and discrimination has upon them to be heard and understood. Many drug users who seek social reintegration have been unable to achieve it. This has not always been due to their own inability to become stable or drug free, but by a 'wall of exclusion,' that has ghettoised problem drug users. The research illustrated how many drug users on Merseyside felt socially stranded, largely forgotten, with little hope or alternatives. It became clear that once a drug using identity is ascribed, no matter how much progress, it is extremely difficult, if not impossible, to overcome the hostile levels of discrimination.

The 200 drug users from across Merseyside involved 134 men and 66 women. The average age was 26 years old and the most common period for drug use was between 7-13 years. In respect of their drug status, 18% said they were currently drug free while a further 58% defined themselves as stable and in control. Most of the sample identified heroin as the drug they were most dependent upon. Just over half had no qualifications whatsoever, and all apart from two people were currently unemployed. One in seven had never had an 'official' job at any point in their life. This discarded working-class group had few legitimate options available to them, and for many, drug taking was an alternative to unemployment, boredom and monotony. As one person stated: *'No prospects for someone like me. I gave up years ago thinking I could get a job, I might as well reach for the moon.'* Many felt that a drug-centred existence was all that was available to them, recognising that it offers an all-consuming alternative, with each day and every day involving the same demanding routine:

a. The person wakes up anxious; concerned about generating sufficient funds to pay for their drug habit and stave off the onset of withdrawal symptoms. For a heroin user around £50 worth of heroin is normally required to get them 'sorted.'
b. Without access to opiates they will soon experience withdrawal symptoms of sickness, stomach cramps, aches, pains and sweating, referred to as 'turkeying.' The first signs are usually experienced soon after the person wakes up.
c. The person then has to set about making plans for the day ahead, providing them with a focus. These plans are almost entirely centred around activities that will generate sufficient funds to enable heroin to be purchased.
d. The person then goes out 'grafting' (committing crime). Any goods stolen will need to be worth considerably more than the cost of the heroin they need to purchase, as they will need to be sold quickly.
e. The stolen goods are sold at a fraction of their true value, often to people living in impoverished communities.
f. With cash in hand after what might be considered a 'hard days work,' the person seeks to purchase some decent quality heroin; this is referred to as going to 'score.'
g. Once they have acquired a 'wrap' of heroin, they find a safe place to enjoy the 'reward' for their hard work, hoping that what they have bought is indeed heroin and doesn't contain any dangerous impurities.

h. At the end of this they can then find some rest or sleep only to begin the same routine for another day–every day.

This isolating existence appears to have had a deep and intrusive impact on the self-esteem of dependent drug users. When asked how they feel about being with people who aren't drug users, many expressed feelings of unworthiness, feelings of being second-class citizens:

> *'They look down on me as scum of the earth and as someone not to be associated with.'*

> *'most people look down their noses at me.'*

> *'they see me as a drug addict, a smackhead and they think I'd rob them.'*

> *'some people think you are scum.'*

In addition other drug users comments illustrated a growing sense of unease and anxiety emerging:

> *'I feel beneath them, they make you feel like that'; 'I feel the odd one out, I've nothing in common with them. I start to get paranoid.'*

> *'I used to avoid them like the plague. I used to be scared of what they might think.'*

> *'I feel nervous in case I slip up, I know they would look at me in disgust.'*

This fear of rejection has led to some drug users feeling they cannot risk being honest:

> *'I feel I have to make up for being on drugs. I have to be at my best, I don't want people to look down on me so I make everything look perfect.'*

This isolation and exclusion perpetuates drug use preventing and hindering opportunities for social reintegration:

> *'I never really mixed with people who have never taken drugs.'*

When asked about the quality of their relationships many drug users had little or no relationships that they would describe as friendships. Instead, they referred to having acquaintances with drug associates that were largely functional:

> *'I had drug associates and only one friend, really.'*

This lonely and dehumanising experience ultimately undermines their ability to form relationships and tends to reinforce social isolation and subsequent dislocation. The harsh and demanding drug-centred lifestyle is, for many, all that is on offer. In the 'normal' world from which they have been excluded many feel vulnerable and lack confidence, and thus the cycle is perpetuated. When asked about why they used drugs it was clear that some used drugs to mask this sense of inadequacy:

> '*I'd use drugs to give me confidence.*'

> '*One of the reasons I use is that I get confidence but it's a false confidence.*'

The war on drugs has failed to recognise the structural factors that have left large sections of society socially and economically stranded. Drug users are portrayed as callous criminals who have little regard for others. However, when asked about their involvement in crime, many committed crimes only to support their drug addiction:

> '*I'm not a thief, I'm not a robber, it's because of the drugs and my situation.*'

> '*I was using street drugs and I had to find money to support my habit.*'

Many who were maintained on methadone or were drug free had managed to remove themselves from the criminal scene altogether:

> '*Now that I'm on a script, I'm not offending; it was only ever to support my habit.*'

> '*I'm not using so I don't need to find money.*'

The underlying factors that create the climate for problematic (not recreational) drug use tend to be structural, and drug use remains much higher in poor neighbourhoods (Foster 2000). Rarely are such factors addressed, indeed treatment agencies are often poorly resourced and dogged by long waiting lists. While millions of UK pounds are spent on drug enforcement, little is allocated to treatment and rehabilitation. A staggering 85% of the UK drug budget is spent upon prevention, prohibition and punishment (European Monitoring Centre for Drugs and Drug Addiction 1997:319) and although the balance is beginning to shift amidst recognition that treatment is under resourced, it will be a long time before a more appropriate balance is achieved. Resources to assist drug users need to be more robust. Although a small proportion of drug users don't want to change their situation, it was clear from these three research studies that many became depressed, tired and frustrated, trapped within a drug-centred life, wanting help to change, but seeing no realistic options available to them.

In the Bootle study (Buchanan & Young 1996), designed to identify the needs of local dependent drug users, when asked to identify the main difficulties they faced as drug users, low self-esteem and poor confidence featured as a major factor (64% of respondents) followed closely by finances and relationship issues. Surprisingly, legal and health issues scored lowest. The qualitative data revealed that confidence and self-esteem are seen by drug users as a crucial factors for recovery:

> *'it doesn't matter about anything else, if you don't have confidence.'*

> *'I need my self-esteem back, it just affects everything.'*

> *'with confidence you've more chance of carrying things out.'*

The action research of the Structured Day Programme 'Transit' (Buchanan & Young 1998a) findings highlighted the importance of social rehabilitation and the need to ensure that core social work values inform practice. When asked about the staff at the Structured Day Programme, drug users identified developing trust and being non-judgemental as key factors:

> *'Most of them [the staff] I got on with. It surprised me. I don't normally trust people.'*

> *'They're non-judgmental.'*

> *'They've all been sound and approachable.'*

A common theme that emerged from the drug users was that many felt inferior and undeserving. The following comments illustrate the extent to which some drug users have internalised an identity as undeserving second class citizens

> *'We're very lucky to have somewhere like this and to be treated like equals.'*

> *'I didn't rate myself doing anything before this has given me hope.'*

THE DEVELOPMENT OF A NEW CONCEPTUAL FRAMEWORK

Contrary to discourses that have emphasised the importance of addressing physiological and psychological aspects of drug dependence, these findings suggest that the social dimension to drug use must be acknowledged, understood and integrated into policies and practices if rehabilitation and reintegration are to become realistic and achievable goals for long term problem drug users. The stage oriented model developed by Prochaska and DiClemente (1982), based originally on helping cigarette smokers quit, has proved extremely effective in helping understand the distinct stages of dependent behaviour. Significantly, the identification of the 'appropriate phase' has enabled drug workers to adopt the most effective and suitable intervention (Barber 1995). Commonly referred to as the 'cycle for change,' it has with good reason dominated UK theory and practice with drug users. Paradoxically, the model has led to a risk that drug workers pathologise clients' drug problems, by concentrating upon individual motivation and psychological strategies for change. These are helpful and important factors but the social context and structural realities faced by problem drug users need to be incorporated. The Steps to Reintegration (Figure 1) attempts to conceptualise the experiences of the drug users involved in the three Merseyside studies, and it seeks to integrate the psychological and the structural:

FIGURE 1

STEPS to REINTEGRATION

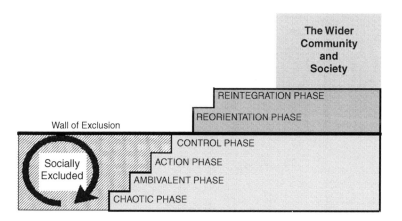

Each phase is discrete and drug users will tend to work their way up the steps one at a time. Some may remain on one step for a long time, others for a short period. It is also possible for leaps (missing steps) to be made upward or downward, though the latter is much more common than the former. Recognising where a drug user is on the steps is crucial as it enables a more appropriate response to be made. Accurate assessment of motivation is often hindered by subtle coercive pressure from agency staff for the drug user to agree to a particular treatment regime. The diagram offers an alternative explanation to the long accepted chronically relapsing nature of drug dependence. Rather than it being the result of psychological dependence, craving or physical addiction, the Steps to Reintegration model suggests it is social exclusion and discrimination that are major factors leading to relapse. Once progress is made and drug users gain control, it is this often-impenetrable 'wall of exclusion' that separates and prevents drug users from re-entering and participating in society. In the three Merseyside studies 76% of the drug users described themselves as either drug free or stable and in control, yet the common experience was that they felt stranded and isolated with a drug subculture, afraid of being with the non-drug-using population, unable to break through the wall of exclusion.

Significantly, the vast majority of services for drug users operate below the wall of exclusion, helping drug users to regain control or become drug free. There are in the UK only a limited number of drug agencies primarily concerned with the reorientation and social reintegration of drug users into mainstream society. Some mainstream agencies concerned with social inclusion do have this role, though their remit is not specifically to assist drug users. However, it is not uncommon for drug users attending such agencies to be treated with suspicion, caution and unease.

INDIVIDUAL STAGES TO INTEGRATION

At the *chaotic phase* problem drug users do not see that they have a problem with drugs, and if they do they are usually unwilling or unable to contemplate change. This stage is often typified by an all-consuming drug-centred existence in which satisfying the need or craving for drugs can override most other issues or concerns. At this stage dependent drug users are unlikely to be able to respond to well-meaning advice, guidance or coercion. Attempts to persuade drug users of the genuine harm or risks they face are usually met with avoidance or with a passive outward acceptance countered by an inward hidden rejection. What is particularly important at this stage is to develop an honest and accepting relationship that gives the drug user permission to communicate what their intentions are in relation to drugs, without the fear of rejection or moralising from the agency worker. Within this relationship it is then possible to offer realistic strategies that may reduce the degree of risk or harm to the drug users, their family or wider community. This could include: accurate information about the risk and effects of drugs, access to clean needles, substitute prescribing on a daily pick-up basis, improvements of injecting technique, etc.

At the *ambivalent phase* the dependent drug user is periodically beginning to acknowledge negative aspects of being dependent on drugs and these feelings cause shifts in their motivation when s/he is contemplating making changes. It would be a mistake at such times, to try and capture one of these moments and exploit the opportunity to the full. This tends to result in a coerced drug user who may initially value the attention and help, obligingly agree to treatment, but soon relapses and then feels guilty for letting the worker down. This is classically referred to as 'setting the drug user up to fail.' When this happens the drug users' confidence and self-esteem can be further damaged as well as their relationship with the worker, whom they may feel they have disappointed and let down. The emphasis required at this stage is to enable the drug user to explore the pros and cons of their pattern of drug use and lifestyle in general. The worker needs to avoid projecting their own personal/professional thinking, values, choices or interpretations, but instead facilitate space for the drug user to explore these issues from *their* perspective. The tension of competing priorities as determined by the individual drug user is much more likely to trigger internal motivation for change than arguments presented by the worker.

At the *action phase* the dependent drug user has already decided what s/he wants to do and is beginning to make preparations for when and how to commence different stages and where to receive additional support. Action does not necessarily mean a decision to become drug free; for example, it could be a decision to move from injecting heroin to smoking it. Most problem drug users are likely to have been dependent for many years, and will already have had a number of unsuccessful attempts to regain control of their drug habit. It is important, therefore, at this phase, that the person pursues assistance appropriate to their need and situation, and at a pace of change that is realistic and manageable. Mistakes can be made either by the drug user or the worker, rushing, enforcing, or pushing change. Anxious to achieve and seize the moment, this sometimes leads to poor planning, such as rushing to the first Drug Rehabilitation Centre that has vacancies rather than carefully considering the most suitable one. Good planning and preparation is crucial, this needs to include viable alternatives to fill any vacuum left by the departure from a busy drug-centred lifestyle.

The *control phase* refers to that period when the dependent drug user has taken the planned action and has successfully regained control of their drug use. This is a time of change and uncertainty for the drug user; they need to begin thinking ahead to what new habits and interests are going to replace the old ones. It is likely too, as the above extracts indicate, that they may be quite apprehensive about the idea of mixing with non-drug users. If their long-term goal is to become completely abstinent they may be worried about meeting old acquaintances or about the onset of unexpected craving. This is a vulnerable period in which the drug user can swing between confidence about staying in control and unpredictable anxiety about possible relapse. It is helpful at this stage to explore and rehearse both the drug user's and agency worker's response to relapse, and to seek to learn positively from it, if or when it occurs. It can be misleading at this stage for the drug user to think that they have resolved their difficulties because they are now in control of their drug consumption; however, as illustrated earlier, the difficulties problem drug users face go beyond physical and psychological dependence. Lifestyle, friendships, daily routines, confidence, self-esteem, health, education, and employment are all issues that will need careful consideration. The likelihood of successful transition will depend heavily upon the drug user's opportunity to move away from a drug centred existence and begin to establish alternative routines and patterns.

The Wall of Exclusion is not a phase but a barrier that makes it extremely difficult for recovering drug users to become accepted into the structures and networks of everyday life. The propaganda designed to deter people from trying illegal drugs by portraying drug users as a deviant enemy has led to a war on drug users themselves. This has resulted in discrimination at every level. For many drug users relapse is not attributable simply to the physical craving or a change in motivation, but as a consequence of their frustration at trying to break into mainstream community life and finding themselves constantly shunned and excluded. At the very time when recovering drug users need assistance and support from the non-drug-using population to establish alternative patterns of social and economic life, they are often prevented by the wall of exclusion.

The *reorientation phase* is a particularly challenging period when the drug user is in control of their habit and trying to actively reorient themselves with new activities, lifestyle patterns and habits away from the drug scene. It is important that the goals and plans here are realistic, achievable and suitable for the drug user. For many problem drug users in the research mentioned earlier, sleeping patterns, finance, education, employment, fitness, diet, and friendship networks had all been seriously undermined. For some this had become a chronic problem:

'I go to bed at 10.30pm and can wake up at 3am and not get back. It can happen at least twice a week. I'm fucked and it pisses me off.'

'Before methadone I couldn't sleep til dawn. I was so tired it was terrible, my mind would be whirring round I just wanted to turn it off.'

'I am not eating regular meals it depends upon my frame of mind as to if I buy food or drugs first.'

'I snacked on crisps and shite.'

'I'm underweight I'm 8st 3lbs–I should be 9stone.'

Confidence and self-esteem are likely to be damaged leaving the drug user vulnerable and in need of regular support and encouragement. Many drug users felt uneasy and threatened in the company of non-drug users, yet this is the group of people whose support, friendship, and integration is crucial. Sheltered environments specifically designed to assist drug users, such as Structured Day Programmes, day centres, befriending or buddying schemes are useful at this stage, but such services are scarce. For a drug user who hasn't eaten three meals a day or slept through the night for the past 6 years (and this wasn't unusual in our studies), the reorientation phase can take a significant amount of time.

The *reintegration phase* is the period when the dependent drug users begin to participate and join in mainstream activities. Due to negative experiences, many drug users feel anxious and afraid of judgmental attitudes from the non-drug-using population, and understandably tend to lack confidence. Normal day-to-day activities such as engaging in further education, doing voluntary work, attending a school meeting, doing a vocational adult education course, joining the local gym can be very intimidating as many have been disconnected from mainstream activities. They face a dilemma of whether to disclose their drug history, knowing that, ironically, honesty is likely to lead to distrust and possible discrimination. Acceptance and belonging within non-drug-using communities will enable the drug user to complete the break from a drug-centred lifestyle. Unless 'doors open' and drug users are sufficiently integrated and purposefully occupied it will be hard to sustain, and the risk of relapse looms. This reintegration phase is crucial if the drug user is to successfully make the transition and participate in the social and economic life of her/his local community.

CONCLUSION

This article has argued that the key issues that drug users face are related to discrimination, isolation, and powerlessness. Those drug users who become

long-term and dependent tend to have been disadvantaged and socially excluded from an early age prior to their taking drugs. For many of these people
an all-consuming drug-centred lifestyle was not the problem, but a solution to
a problem. Social work has a long standing tradition of highlighting injustice,
discrimination and inequality, and seeking to empower the service user. Social
workers are then, ideally, placed to make a significant contribution to draw attention and develop increasing awareness and understanding to the issues of
oppression and discrimination that many drug users experience. This is not to
suggest that some drug users don't warrant adverse reactions, but it is to argue
that blanket discrimination is unacceptable. Drug users deserve to be treated as
individuals. Rarely has this happened and many drug users have internalised
the ascribed negative identities which have only served to further damage their
self-worth, and hinder their progress.

The Social work values (www.basw.co.uk) of human rights, empowerment, respect for diversity, respect for the person, fair access to public services, equal treatment, self-determination are particularly relevant when
working with drug users. When agency staff have worked to these values
drug users have noticed the difference and spoken positively of these workers. If the drugs 'problem' is going to be successfully tackled then the wall of
exclusion, which is partly constructed and maintained through tabloid shock
horror campaigns and populist government propaganda, will need removing.
The emphasis on individually pathologising the drug problem through physiological approaches enforced through drug testing or cognitive behavioural
programmes as a condition of Probation Orders needs to be balanced by
strategies and services for drug users that acknowledge the present day social context. The structural dimension to drug dependence must be understood and tackled if genuine progress is to be achieved. The Steps to
Reintegration model offers an alternative paradigm that conceptualises the
notion of discrimination and exclusion. It also enables social work to begin
to focus attention upon addressing the gap in the services by promoting
structured day programmes, day centres, befriending schemes, and sheltered
workshops.

Challenging discrimination is part of the social workers commitment to
Anti-Discriminatory Practice. It is perhaps easier to deliver when society more
readily understands and accepts the issues involved, for example, combating
discrimination that is directed at older people or the discrimination directed at
people with disabilities. However, challenging discrimination towards drug
users attracts little support or sympathy. But then challenging racism or sex-
ism 50 years ago may not have gained much support or sympathy either.

REFERENCES

Advisory Council On The Misuse Of Drugs (1988) AIDS and Drug Misuse Part 1, HMSO, London.

Bandura, A (1977) Social Learning Theory. Englewood Cliffs, N.J.: Prentice-Hall

Barber JG (1995) Social Work with Addictions Macmillan Press London

Beck A (1979) Cognitive Therapy and the Emotional Disorders, NAL Books, New York

British Association of Social Workers Web Site (2002) www.basw.co.uk

Buchanan J & Young L (1996) Drug Relapse Prevention: Giving Users a Voice Bootle Maritime City Challenge, Liverpool

Buchanan J & Young L (1998) 'Failing To Grasp The Nettle: UK Drug Policy' Probation Journal Vol. 45 No. 4

Buchanan J & Young L (1998a) The Impact Of The Second Chance Structured Day Programme for Recovering Drug Users: A Student Perspective Liverpool, Social Partnership, Transit

Buchanan J & Young L (2000) 'The War on Drugs; A War on Drug Users' Drugs: Education Prevention & Policy, Vol. 7 No.4 2000 pp 409-422

Christie, N (1986) 'Suitable Enemies' in Bianchi H & van Swaaningen R (eds), Abolitionistm: Towards a Non-repressive Approach to Crime. Amsterdam: Free University Press pp. 42-54

Christie, N & Bruun K (1985) *Den gode fiende. Narkotikapolitikk i Norden.* (The useful enemy. Drug-policy in the Nordic countries) Universitetsforlaget, Ejlers. Oslo/Copenhagen

Department of Health (2001) Statistical Bulletin 2001/33, Statistics from the Regional Drug Misuse Databases on Drug Misusers in Treatment in England, 2000/01, Office for National Statistics, 2001

Drucker E (2000) 'From Morphine to Methadone; Maintenance Drugs in the Treatment of Opiate Addiction' in Harm Reduction National and International Perspectives, Incardia J A & Harrison L D (eds) Sage, London

European Monitoring Centre for Drugs and Drug Addiction (1999) Extended Annual Report of the Drug Problem in the European Union, Lisbon, EMCDDA

Foster J (2000) 'Social Exclusion Crime and Drugs' Drugs Education, Prevention, and Policy Vol 7 No. 4 pp 317-330

Goldson B, Kennedy J & Young L (1995) Second Chance Opportunities: A Service Users Perspective, Liverpool Drug Prevention Initiative

Hansard (1990) House of Commons Debates 25th January 1990 Column 864, HMSO, London

Hartnoll R (1998) 'International trends in Drug Policy' in The Control of Drugs and Drug Users Reason or Reaction? Coomber R Harwood Academic Publishers, Amsterdam

Her Majesty's Government (1998) Tackling Drugs to Build a Better Britain Cm 3945, The Stationery Office, London

HM Treasury (2001) £300 Million Boost For Communities Against Drugs, Press Release, 49/01 09 April 2001

Lancet Editorial (2001) Rethinking America's "War on Drugs" as a public health issue Vol. 357, No. 9261, p 971 31 March 2001

May T, Harocopos A, Turnbull P & Hough M (2000) Serving Up: The Impact of Low-Level Police Enforcement on Drug Markets, Home Office, London

McDermott P (2001) 'Reflections on British Drug Policy,' conference paper presented at the 1st UK Harm Reduction Alliance, Conference, Blackpool

Measham F, Aldridge J & Parker H (2001) Dancing on Drugs; Risk, Health, and Hedonism in the British Club Scene, Free Association Books, London

Miller W & Rollnick S (1991) Motivational Interviewing, Guilford Press, London

Murji K (1998) Policing Drugs, Ashgate, Aldershot

Parker H, Aldridge J & Measham J (1998) Illegal Leisure, Routledge, London

Police Foundation (2000) Drugs and the Law. Report of the Independent Inquiry into the Misuse of Drugs Act 1971, Police foundation, London

Prochaska JO & DiClemente C.C (1982) 'Transtheoretical Therapy: Towards a More Integrated Model of Change' Psychotherapy, 20, pp 161-173

Prochaska JO, DiClemente CC, & Norcross, JC (1992). In Search of How People Change. Applications to Addictive Behaviors. *American Psychologist, 47,* 1102-1113

Ramsay M & Partridge S (1999) Drug Misuse Declared in 1998: Results from the British Crime Survey, London, Home Office

Riley D & O'Hare P (2000) 'Harm Reduction: History, Definition, and Practice' in Incardia J & Harrison L Harm Reduction National and International Perspectives, Sage Publications, London

Robson P (1999) Forbidden Drugs, second edition, Oxford University Press, Oxford

Royal College of Psychiatrists (2001) Drugs Dilemmas & Choices Gaskell, London

South N (1997) 'Drug Use, Crime, and Control' in The Oxford Handbook of Criminology Second Edition, Maguire M, Morgan R, & Reiner R (eds) Clarendon Press, Oxford

Thompson N (2001) Anti-Discriminatory Practice, Third Edition, Basingstoke, Palgrave

Trebach A (1987) The Great Drug War: And Radical Proposal That Could Make America Safe Again, MacMillan Press

United Nations Office for Drug Control and Crime Prevention UNDCCP (1997) World Drug Report, Oxford University Press, Oxford

U.S. Department of Justice (2001) Bureau of Justice Statistics Bulletin Prisoners in 2000 August 2001, CJ 188207

Van Ree E (1997) 'Fear of Drugs' International Journal of Drug Policy, 8 (2) pp 93-100

Walmsley R (2000) World Prison Population List, 2nd Edition, Research Findings No. 116, Home Office, London

Community Care in Taiwan: Mere Talk, No Policy

Yueh-Ching Chou
Teppo Kröger

SUMMARY. This article explores the policy definitions and the funder roles of central and local governments in community care in Taiwan. The notion of community care has been adopted in Taiwan following the model of Hong Kong but the main question of the article is whether this has resulted in actual service provisions at the community level, forming an alternative to institutional care. The data has been collected from several sources: policy documents, official statistics, surveys, general reports, funding provision reports, and empirical studies. The results show that neither central nor local authorities are seriously involved in caring for elderly people or persons with disabilities in Taiwan's communities. In Taiwan, community care for these groups of people still means, in practice, informal care provided by female family members without any support from public policies. *[Article copies available for a fee from The Haworth Document Delivery Service: 1-800-HAWORTH. E-mail address: <docdelivery@haworthpress.com> Website: <http://www.HaworthPress.com> © 2004 by The Haworth Press, Inc. All rights reserved.]*

Yueh-Ching Chou, PhD, is Associate Professor, Institute of Health and Welfare Policy, National Yang-Ming University, 155, Li-Nong Street, Sec. 2, Peitou, Taipei, Taiwan (Email: choucyc@ym.edu.tw).

Teppo Kröger, PhD, is Lecturer, Department of Social Sciences and Philosophy, University of Jyväskylä, Jyväskylä, Finland (E-mail: teppo.kroger@yfi.jyu.fi).

[Haworth co-indexing entry note]: "Community Care in Taiwan: Mere Talk, No Policy." Chou, Yueh-Ching and Teppo Kröger. Co-published simultaneously in *Social Work in Mental Health* (The Haworth Social Work Practice Press, an imprint of The Haworth Press, Inc.) Vol. 2, No. 2/3, 2004, pp. 139-156; and: *Social Work Approaches in Health and Mental Health from Around the Globe* (ed: Metteri et al.) The Haworth Social Work Practice Press, an imprint of The Haworth Press, Inc., 2004, pp. 139-156. Single or multiple copies of this article are available for a fee from The Haworth Document Delivery Service [1-800-HAWORTH, 9:00 a.m. - 5:00 p.m. (EST). E-mail address: docdelivery@haworthpress.com].

KEYWORDS. Community care, care in the community, care by the community, family care, disability, elderly, carer

INTRODUCTION

Community care is a new concept in Taiwan. It was used for the first time in Taipei City in 1995 referring to a special approach that was used in an experiment in working with elderly and disabled people. The arrival of the concept to Taiwan dates back to two years earlier, year 1993, when a conference on "Community Care in the Chinese Society" was held in Hong Kong (Chen, 1995; Su, 1995).

However, there is still no clear understanding about what is meant by community care in Taiwan. It is usually referred to as an intervention approach in working with disabled people and the elderly but there is no clearly agreed definition of it among practitioners. On the other hand, government documents refer to the concept in a broader sense but, in addition, they use a Taiwanese concept of "welfare communitilization," not making a distinctive separation between these two.

Thus, the status of community care within social policy in Taiwan is far from clear. This paper sets out to clarify the situation first by asking how community care is defined in Taiwanese social policy documents. This will be followed by an even more significant question: Do there actually exist policies and service programs regarding care in the community in Taiwan? What are the roles of central and local governments in supporting the everyday life of elderly and disabled people at the community level? Do there really exist functioning community care policies in Taiwan or is the talk about community care just a new discourse for the old approach of inaction? Answers to these questions are sought by collecting and analyzing official statistics (1998, 1999, and 1999/2000), survey reports, earlier studies, and governmental documents including white papers, inspection, service, and funding provision reports.

These empirical parts about Taiwan are preceded by a short review of community care literature in Britain and Hong Kong.

REVIEW OF LITERATURE FROM BRITAIN AND HONG KONG

The concept of community care was adopted to Taiwan from Hong Kong and in Hong Kong, as its former colony, policy discussions have been influenced by social policies practiced in Britain. Even in Britain, the definitions and policies of community care are not consistent (Walker, 1982, 1989; Maclean,

1989; Ramon, 1991; Davis & Ellis, 1995; Tester, 1996; Clements, 1996, 1997). Nevertheless, the main goal of care in the community is in Britain to provide an alternative to institutionalization (Titmuss, 1968; Walker, 1981; Payne, 1986; Hunter & Wistow, 1987, 1989; Cooper, 1989; Ramom, 1991). This requires the development of a wide range of services provided in the community setting (DHSS, UK, 1989, p. 9). As a result, "care in the community" stands in the British discussion for a variety of locally provided de-institutionalized care services, aimed to enable people to live in their homes (or in "homely settings") and achieve as much independence and control over their own lives as possible.

However, in the British administrative context, the term "community care service" is often used to refer to most of the services provided by the social service departments of local authorities, including also residential social services (Mandelstam, 1998). In addition to social care provided by local governments, primary health care provided by national health authorities is usually counted as community care (DHSS, UK, 1989). Community care services are addressed also to people with physical or mental disabilities but there is no doubt that the main user group in Britain is elderly people (Audit Commission, UK, 1986; Baggott, 1994). Since the 1980s, there has been continuous discussion in Britain about whether emphasis should be moved from providing formal services, that is, from "care in the community" to "care by the community," to enable and promote informal care by families and social networks. Critiques to this proposed policy change have said that focusing on "care by the community" implicates leaving care responsibilities solely to female carers in the households (Segal, 1979; McCarthy, 1989; Walker, 1989, 1997; Sainsbury, 1995).

In Hong Kong, the term "care in the community" was used for the first time in governmental documents in 1973 in a report that sketched new directions for services for elderly people (Chow, 1988). Accordingly, in Hong Kong community care means predominately elderly care in the community. Community care services include community support services such as domiciliary care, home help, and meal services but also residential services (Lee, 1993).

The concept of community care was adopted to Hong Kong from Britain but based on specific historical and cultural contexts, interpretations of "care in the community" and "care by the community" are different in Britain and Hong Kong. For Hong Kong, community care means mostly family care (1965 White Paper "Aims and Policy for Social Welfare in Hong Kong"; Social Welfare into the 1990s and Beyond–White Paper, Hong Kong Government, 1991; 1994 Report Working Group On Care for the Elderly, Hong Kong). Kan (1993) and Wang (1990), two professionals working in Hong Kong, transformed the British concepts of "care by the community" and "care in the community" into "community organization" and "community work." According to their interpretations, "care in the community" means moving the place of care from institutions into the community, "community" being here a geographical concept. On the other hand, "care by the community" means that service users are cared for by family members, relatives, friends, neighbors, volunteers, and professionals working in the community; here "community" is a functional concept.

Hence, professionals in Hong Kong utilize community work and strive to improve "community supportive networks," "care networks," and "close community relationships" (Lee, 1987; Kan, 1993; Su, 1994a). Under this framework of promoting mutual-help community relationships, dependent persons are expected to be cared for by the networks living in the community, including family members but also voluntary organizations, churches, and neighbors (1977 Green Paper "Services for the Elderly" in Hong Kong). The methods of community development and community organization are the main strategies to facilitate the residents' involvement in care-giving in the community (Shu, 1980, 1985; Tung, 1971; Su, 1996). The aims of community care policies in Hong Kong are "to allow the elderly to be cared for in and by the community" (1980 The Five Year Plan for Social Welfare Development in Hong Kong–Review 1980), "to foster the concept of old people as an integrated part of the community, and to promote mutual understanding between young and old" (1985 The Five Year Plan for Social Welfare Development in Hong Kong–Review 1985), and, finally, to make "aging in place" a synonym for "care in the community" (1994 Report Working Group on Care for the Elderly, Hong Kong). In all, policies wish to promote the building of a caring community.

Not all meanings of community care related concepts are fully clear and shared in Hong Kong (Yeung, 1992; Chow, 1993; Kan, 1995; Huang & Chen, 1996), nor are they in Britain. However, it is evident that Hong Kong concentrates mainly on upholding the caring capacity of local communities whereas Britain has constructed a network of formal social and health care services with extensive regional coverage. In 1993, the concept of community care was adopted to Taiwan from Hong Kong but what meanings does the concept carry in Taiwan? Are the interpretations of "care in the community" and "care by the community" different from those in Britain or Hong Kong?

DEFINITIONS OF COMMUNITY CARE IN TAIWAN

Following definitions from Hong Kong, Su has defined community care in Taiwan as a linkage between formal and informal systems, including also voluntary and family systems. Community care in Taiwan aims to provide care services to the needy in their own homes or in the community enabling them to have "a normal life" and to enhance their ability of living and integrating with the community. As in Hong Kong, community care is to build a caring community (Su, 1994b, p. 55, 1995, p. 65; Kan, 1993).

The approaches of community care promoted in the Taiwanese literature include case management (Lou, 1998) and community work, focusing especially on community organization and networking with voluntary organizations (Su, 1996; Lou, 1996). On the other hand, community care has also been identified as long-term care for the disabled elderly, providing institutional care, home nursing care, and welfare services in the community (Shieh & Lieu, 1996; Shieh, 1997). Su (1994a, 1994b, 1996) and Chen (1995) have emphasized that "care in the community" is equated and intertwined with "care by the community" in Taiwan, the former concept highlighting the place of care and the latter concept favoring a close connection between voluntary providers and central and local governments.

Based on these definitions and concepts, community care is understood in the literature in Taiwan as care of those dependent persons, mainly persons with severe disabilities and the frail elderly, who live with their families and who are cared for in the community. From the perspective of the families, the main question is whether community care means pure family care or, instead, intra-/extra-family care systems that include support from voluntary and professional sources outside the family. The literature from Taiwan seems to back the latter alternative. As a result, community organization and community work have been presented as important approaches in order to motivate the community's mutual support for persons with severe disabilities and the disabled elderly (Su, 1995, 1996).

However, these discussions within the literature written by scholars and practitioners are not fully reflected in public policies in Taiwan. On the contrary, the concept of community care has not been used in the main policy documents from central government. In particular, the most important social welfare policy document in Taiwan– "The Principles of Social Welfare Policy and Programs of 1994," published by the Executive Yuan, that is, the Office of the Premier–does not even mention community care. It only states that it is the government's role to develop family-centered welfare services in order to promote Chinese family ethics, and to use community organization as a method to develop welfare services in the community.

However, following the direction of this principle document, the Ministry of Interior, which is the highest social welfare bureaucracy in Taiwan, declared in 1996 a program of "Improving Social Welfare Communitilization: Directions of Implementation." With this plan the Ministry brought in a concept of their own, "welfare communitilization," thus avoiding the need to take community care as the prime term. The Ministry stated that the goal of "welfare communitilization" is to use community work as a method to establish linkages with non-governmental resources from voluntary, informal, and commercial sectors. Furthermore, the document recommended that welfare services should be improved by changing over to smaller institutional care units (Harris & Chou, 2001).

As a result, the terms "welfare communitilization" and "community care" are often used interchangeably and in a mixed way in Taiwan (Harris & Chou, 2001). For instance, "welfare communitilization" has been written as "community care" in several official documents (Welfare Subvention Regulations for Promoting Social Welfare in 2000; the Welfare Subvention Programs and Standards for Promoting Social Welfare in 2000, Department of Social Affairs, Ministry of Interior, ROC, 2000a, 2000b). Some authors (Won, 1998; Chang & Wang, 1999) have explained that "welfare communitilization" equals to "local care" and "local services." According to national policy documents, the term "community care" is strictly reserved for disability and elderly welfare services. It is usually understood as home help and respite care services for the elderly and persons with disabilities (1997 Protection Act of Persons with Disabilities, Article 40 & 41; 1997 the Elderly Welfare Act, Article 18; Welfare Subvention Programs and Standards for Promoting Social Welfare in 2000, pp. 54-55).

Concerning local governmental documents, the "White Paper of Taipei Government" from 1994 Taipei City Government used terms such as "intensification, de-institutionalization, decentralization, and communitilization of social welfare systems," emphasizing the implementation of community network services for elderly and disabled people. Five years later, the capital made an interpretation that community care for the elderly includes the provision of home help services, nursing care services at home, day care services, agency-based respite care services, and improving the home living environment (Taipei City Government, 1999). Other local authorities in Taiwan have no document defining the term community care in their local areas. They merely follow the central governmental documents, in order to apply for a grant from the Ministry of Interior.

As a result, at the local level, it is only Taipei City Government that has self used the term "community care" and given it a definition of providing welfare services to its elderly population. In Taipei City community care is understood as family supportive services, excluding institutional care. This is in line with the afore-mentioned central governmental documents, and these interpretations have been used also by the three other local authorities.

In governmental documents in Taiwan, "welfare communitilization" has thus a broader meaning than what "community care" has. The former term is used by the central government and it includes institutional care that is provided in the community. The latter term is used to describe the family supportive services of local authorities–in practice, this means home help services for the elderly and respite care services for carers of persons with disabilities. At both administrative levels, the concepts of "community care" and "welfare communitilization" are quite new and they are not used in a perfectly unambiguous way.

Following the central governmental plan from 1996, Young (1997), Chen (1997), Su (1998), and Chen (1998) have argued that the essence of "welfare communitilization" is reducing the size of institutions. Accordingly, instead of concentrating on non-institutional services, policies in Taiwan concentrate on institutional care, on making the institutions smaller in size and more integrated into the community. Consequently, concerning welfare communitilization or community care in Taiwan, central government is mostly concerned about geography, bed size of care institutions, and about building resources and networks with volunteers and non-governmental organizations. On the other hand, this means that in Taiwan the state has not planned community care to be an alternative to institutionalization. According to policy documents, community care in Taiwan is a mixed group of services that are of secondary importance to central authorities and that have been left to the responsibility of local authorities.

Next, we will analyze the expenditure figures of central and local governments in Taiwan, particularly spending on community care services.

PUBLIC SPENDING ON COMMUNITY CARE IN TAIWAN

First, if we look at the investment level of central government of Taiwan on elderly and disability welfare, we can see that it has remained quite constant during the fiscal years of 1998, 1999, and 1999-2000 (1.5 years). The shares of these two sectors from the funding of the whole social welfare have been rather stable (Table 1). In addition to being rather unchanged, the spending level of central authorities on the welfare of elderly and disabled people is low: only about 1% of the welfare budget is spent on elderly people and 2-3% on disabled people. Even though the share of disabled people is bigger, both of these two groups receive only a minor slice of the total budget.

However, when the internal division of these slices is looked at, there are huge differences between elderly and disabled people. At least half of the central governmental budget on the welfare of elderly people has been used on non-institutional community care services. The main spending targets within this column have been recreation centers and leisure activities (varying from

TABLE 1. Central Government Budget for Social Welfare of Elderly and Disabled People in Taiwan in 1998, 1999, and 1999-2000*

Year	Elderly/ social welfare (%)	Community care/ elderly (%)	Disability/ Social welfare (%)	Community care/ disability (%)
1998	1.1	48.9	2.4	1.1
1999	1.1	47.9	2.6	1.0
1999-2000	0.8	65.6	2.1	1.1

*1998: 1 year, 1999: 1 year, 1999-2000: 1 1/2 years.
Source: Fiscal budget plans on social welfare by the Ministry of Interior of ROC, 1998, 1999, 1999-2000.

18.0 to 22.2% of the elderly welfare budget), day care services (13.3%-15.8%) and home help services (5.4%-10.7%). In the fiscal year 1999-2000, also an attendance allowance and a care subsidy for low-income families were included in the community care expenditure for elderly people.

Instead, the division of social welfare funds for the care of disabled people has been totally different. Only 1% of all central government disability funding has been used on community care services such as home help and respite care. In other words, central authorities in Taiwan spend practically their full disability budget on institutional care. Some central funds are used on a means- and needs-tested family care allowance ("Living with Family Subsidy"). Its receivers are not allowed to use care services such as day care or institutional care.

Second, we will look at the spending levels of local governments. Here, data is gathered from four of 22 local authorities in Taiwan: the capital Taipei City, Tainan City, Chang-hwa County, and Yi-lan County. First, their spending on elderly people is presented (Table 2).

There are disparities between the different Taiwanese local authorities in their social welfare spending. Generally local authorities have mostly spent between 15% and 30% of their welfare budgets on elderly people even though there are some surprisingly large yearly fluctuations, explained probably by changes in statistical practices. In one local authority (Yi-lan County) this share has been up to 60%.

There are also variations in the budget shares that these local authorities spend on community care for elderly people. In the capital Taipei City, around one quarter of the elderly budget is used on non-institutional services such as transportation (which takes a major part, 15-20% of the whole elderly budget), home help, day care, and recreation activities. In Tainan City, this figure has remained around 10% mostly as a result of supporting the transportation of elderly people only slightly and emphasizing recreational activities instead. On the other hand, Chang-hwa County has used a third of its elderly budget in 1998 and 1999 on community care, also here the main spending targets being recreation and leisure. Out of the four local authorities, Yi-lan County has invested the smallest share in non-institutional services for older people.

Concerning the expenditures on services for disabled people, there are variations between local authorities in Taiwan as well (Table 3). In this respect,

TABLE 2. Local Government Budgets for Social Welfare of Elderly People in Taipei City, Tainan City, Chang-hwa County, and Yi-lan County in 1998, 1999, and 1999-2000*

Year	Taipei City		Tainan City		Chang-hwa County		Yi-lan County	
	Elderly/ social welfare (%)	Community care/ elderly (%)	Elderly/ social welfare (%)	Community care/ elderly (%)	Elderly/ social welfare (%)	Community care/ elderly (%)	Elderly/ social welfare (%)	Community care/ elderly (%)
1998	29.9	15.5	20.4	11.2	12.4	30.5	58.9	2.7
1999	16.9	28.0	25.9	8.1	6.7	35.9	58.6	5.6
1999-2000	16.1	23.0	64.6	9.0	19.2	13.1	60.6	5.1

* 1998: 1 year, 1999: 1 year, 1999-2000: 11/2 years.

Sources: Fiscal budget plans on social welfare by Taipei City Government, 1998, 1999, 1999-2000; Tainan City Government, 1998, 1999, 1999-2000; Chang-hwa County Government, 1998, 1999, 1999-2000; and Yi-lan County Government, 1998, 1999, 1999-2000.

TABLE 3. Local Government Budgets for Social Welfare of Disabled People in Taipei City, Tainan City, Chang-hwa County, and Yi-lan County in 1998, 1999 and 1999-2000*

Year	Taipei City		Tainan City		Chang-hwa County		Yi-lan County	
	Disability/ social welfare (%)	Community care/ disability (%)	Disability/ social welfare (%)	Community care/ disability (%)	Disability/ social welfare (%)	Community care/ disability (%)	Disability/ social welfare (%)	Community care/ disability (%)
1998	26.1	0.3	4.8	0.0	19.3	0.0	11.5	0.0
1999	27.1	0.3	8.3	0.1	20.6	0.0	16.8	0.0
1999-2000	26.7	0.2	10.6	0.6	26.3	0.6	8.2	0.0

* 1998: 1 year, 1999: 1 year, 1999-2000: 1½ years.

Sources: Fiscal budget plans on social welfare by Taipei City Government, 1998, 1999, 1999-2000; Tainan City Government, 1998, 1999, 1999-2000; Chang-hwa County Government, 1998, 1999, 1999-2000; and Yi-lan County Government, 1998, 1999, 1999-2000.

two local authorities (Taipei City and Chang-hwa County) spend around a quarter of their social welfare budgets on disabled people but the two others spend instead only about a tenth of their welfare expenditure in disability welfare.

Nevertheless, when the internal division of disability funds is concerned, there is an extraordinary resemblance between all the four local authorities. None of them invests practically any funds in non-institutional services for disabled people. The highest figures come from Tainan City and Chang-hwa County from the last financial year, but even then respite care and other community care activities were funded with only 0.6% of the disability welfare budget. One of the local authorities (Yi-lan County) has never set a budget for non-institutional care services for people with disability.

When the funding of community care by both central and local governments is considered at the same time, some general observations can be made. Until the last fiscal year 1999-2000, the volume of central funding for elderly welfare was below the funding level from Taipei City alone. However, the central state has generally invested a larger share of its elderly welfare budget on non-institutional services and also put in a little larger amount of money than what the local authorities have done. Central funds have mostly been used on recreation and day care whereas local funds have been spent on transportation, recreation, day care and home help for low-income families. However, it needs to be remembered that altogether only 0.5% of the total social welfare budget of central authorities has been used in community care for elderly people, whereas the same percentage in the four local authorities has during the three fiscal years varied between 1.6% and 5.8%. In practice, the activity of local governments is a decisive factor as it has been up to them to apply the necessary grants from central government and to actually provide the services. Nevertheless, it must be emphasized that within the social welfare budgets of both levels of authorities, community care for older people is only of a very minor importance.

However, public funding on non-institutional care for elderly people appears as generous if it is compared with the funding for the same services for disabled people. Generally, central authorities put more money in disability than in aging. The share of disability welfare budget out of the total social welfare budget has been at least double the resources of elderly welfare. Also at the local level the resources for disabled people have surpassed the resources for elderly people in Chang-hwa County, and from 1999 in Taipei City, as well. In the two other local authorities the situation has been the opposite. However, the general share of central and local resources that are used to promote the welfare of disabled people is not the real issue here. The real issue is that as well at the central level as at the local level, almost none of the disability funds are used for non-institutional services. Out of the central governmental disability welfare budget, only 1% has been used to fund community care. This lack of central funding has not been compensated by generous funding from the local authorities, on the contrary. None of the four local authorities invest practically anything in community care for disabled people.

FAMILIES BEARING THE RESPONSIBILITY FOR CARE IN TAIWAN

As community care services are so limited for the elderly population and non-existent for the disabled population, how and by whom are they cared for in Taiwan? Is there a large group of elderly and disabled people living in institutions? According to a 1996 survey by the Taiwan government, 85% of the elderly live with their families, 64% with their children and 21% with their spouses. Further 12% of the elderly live alone. Thus, according to this survey, 97% of the elderly in Taiwan live at home and in the community. Only 0.9% were found to live in nursing homes (Statistics Department, Ministry of Interior, ROC, 1996). Concerning people with disabilities, 7.5% of them are in institutional care and 92.5% live in the community, half of all disabled people living alone (Statistics Department, Ministry of Interior, ROC, 2000).

Thus, less than 1% of elderly people and 8 percent of people with disabilities are cared for in institutions and over 90% of the whole elderly and disabled population live in their own homes. It is therefore evident that "care in the community" is reality for the absolute majority of elderly and disabled people in Taiwan. However, instead of receiving community care services from the local governments or the state, they are cared for by informal carers.

Who are these informal caregivers in Taiwan? The main carers of persons with disabilities are their family members including their spouses (15.0%), their mothers (10.2%), their daughters-in-law and daughters (4.8%), sons (3.0%), fathers (2.0%), brothers (0.9%), sisters (0.5%), and other relatives (2.2%). A Taipei City Survey found that 60% of family carers of persons with disabilities are female, particularly spouses and mothers (Fu, Chou, Houng, & Chen, 2000). According to a government survey from 1998, 53% of 15- to 64-year-old female adults are not working, and one third of them have to take care of their dependent family members (Ministry of Interior, ROC, 1998). This means that 17% of all women of working age in Taiwan are full-time, no-pay, family carers for their family members including the elderly and persons with disabilities.

The dominance of family care is based on a strong cultural legacy in Taiwan. The Chinese culture that is grounded on Confucian ideology values

elderly people and relationships between parents and children. Eighty-six percent of Taiwanese people agreed in a survey that taking care of elderly parents is
the responsibility of their children (Leu, 1995). Another national survey showed
that nearly 90% of the elderly see living with their children as the best choice for
their aging and care needs (*http://www.moi.gov.tw/W3/ stat/topic/topic123.html*,
Ministry of Interior, ROC, 2000/1/25). Up till now, leaving parents to live in an
institution has been seen as shameful by both old-age parents and their adult children. In addition, long-term institutional care is too expensive for most families to
use. Central and local governments take responsibility only for those elderly and
disabled people who come from low-income families and who pass financial
means-testing. As a result, the majority of the elderly and disabled people who
live in institutions or nursing homes are from low-income families.

Family care has been promoted also by public policies and legislation. Based
on the Citizen Law, children have duties and responsibilities to maintain their
parents. If they don't carry out these duties, they can be prosecuted. Furthermore, the above-mentioned influential welfare program from 1994 emphasized
precisely "improving Chinese family ethics" (The Principles of Social Welfare
Policy and Programs of 1994, the Executive Yuan, ROC). In linking government and voluntary organizations and in combining their resources at the community level, the main purpose of "welfare communitilization" and "community
care" policies in Taiwan has been to maintain family caring functions. Public
responsibility is limited to disabled and aged people who either are from
low-income families or who don't have a family at all. As a result, the laws and
policies in Taiwan assign family carers the primary role and the overwhelming
responsibility for the care of elderly and disabled people.

DISCUSSION

The concept of community care was adopted to Taiwan from Hong Kong
only a decade ago. In both contexts, community care has been understood to
focus on approaches of community development and case management in order to build resource networks in the community for caring of dependent persons (Lee, 1987; Su, 1994a; Kan, 1993). Since the 1996 central governmental
document, community care has been defined in Taiwan as the goal of "welfare
communitilization" and since then these two terms have been used interchangeably by practitioners and academics. However, community care has
mostly been understood only as a working method with elderly and disabled
persons. Instead, community care has not become a formal policy of the central government. "Welfare communitilization" has been mostly concerned
with reforming institutional care, not in developing an alternative to it. Care

institutions still take the most of the public money that is available to enhance the welfare of elderly and, particularly, disabled people. However, generally people set no value on institutional care, and it is not even available to other than poor families or persons without a family. Some public money is also spent on family care allowances for low-income people but then, these people are excluded from using supportive services.

There is some provision of non-institutional care services for elderly people, mostly by voluntary organizations. Central and local authorities cover the most part of the costs of these activities. However, the provisions are so scarce that at the moment volunteers or professionals are not a real alternative that is available to share the responsibility of family carers. So far, community care can be described as having meant in Taiwan mere talk, no money and no policy. Community care in Taiwan is not actually concerned about elderly and disabled people having opportunities for independent life, but it is only a new term for the old practice of inaction.

Care of elderly and disabled people is still assigned to family members, that is, mostly to women in Taiwan. This is in accordance of the traditional Chinese culture, supported by policies such as the 1994 welfare scheme. The ideology behind public policies is to use "welfare familiarization in order to improve family ethics." Confucianism places a significant value on family responsibility–self help first, before seeking others' help (Wang, 1998).

Also in Britain, community care policies have since the 1980s focused on promoting "care by the community" (Walker, 1982; Meteyard, 1994). However, there this policy has been implemented in addition to–not instead of–developing and upholding an extensive network of publicly funded care services. In Hong Kong the situation is similar to Taiwan in the respect that community care is in practice family care by women (Hu, 1995; Ngan & Wong, 1995). In Hong Kong, however, a larger sphere of voluntary services supports family care and these services receive more generous subvention from the government than in Taiwan. Nevertheless, the main motivation to promote "welfare communitilization" in Taiwan is not to make savings in the central governmental budget, but the government sees it as a way of valuing Chinese culture and rebuilding family function.

International trends have for several decades been away from institutional care and towards community care. However, in the context of Taiwan, if international forces promote de-institutionalization, they may encourage the government to disclaim even the limited responsibility for care of elderly and disabled people that it is currently taking. Community care in Taiwan is still in an experimental stage, and families are still required to take on the lion's share of care responsibilities. Before providing non-institutional community care services has become adopted as a substantial part of social policy by the government, efforts to decrease institutional care will only result in ever more responsibility being pushed to family members.

Will central and local governments in Taiwan ever make such a policy change? The strength of traditional Chinese family values reduces the likelihood of central and local authorities starting to provide and fund non-institutional care services in a large scale. However, also in Taiwan, general trends of social change are building up pressures for the need to rethink care policies. The structures and functions of families are under change. The population is aging and female labor force participation is rising. As a consequence, families in Taiwan will, in the near future, not be able to handle their care responsibilities in the way they have traditionally done. When the care needs are going up and the care capacity of families is going down, authorities will face the necessity to find new solutions.

REFERENCES

In English

Audit Commission, UK. (1986). *Making a reality of community care*. UK: HMSO.
Baggott, R. (1994). *Health and health care in Britain*. London: St. Martin's Press.
Chow, N. (1993). The changing responsibilities of the state and family toward elders in Hong Kong. *Journal of Aging & Social Policy, 5*(1/2), 111-126.
Clements, L. (1997). Community care–Towards a workable statute. *The Liverpool Law Review, 19*(2), 181-191.
Clements, L. (1996). *Community care and the law*. London: Legal Action Group.
Cooper, J. (1989). From casework to community care: 'The end is where we start from' (T. S. Eliot). *British Journal of Social Work, 19*, 177-188.
Davis, A., & Ellis, K. (1995). Enforced altruism in community care. In R. Hugman & D. Smith (Eds.), *Ethical issues in social work* (pp. 136-154). London: Routledge.
Harris, J., & Chou, Y.C. (2001). Globalization or glocalization? Community care in Taiwan and Britain. *European Journal of Social Work, 4*(2), 161-172.
Hunter, D. J., & Wistow, G. (1987). *Community care in Britain: Variations on a theme*. London: King's Found Publishing Office.
Hunter, D. J., & Wistow, G. (1989). Community care policies: Their evolution. In D. J. Hunter & G. Wistow (Eds.), *Acting on the agenda: Principles and responsibilities in community care* (pp. 5-9). Leeds: The Nuffield Institute for Health Services Studies, University of Leeds.
Maclean, U. (1989). *Dependent territories: The frail elderly and community care*. London: The Nuffield Provincial Hospitals Trust.
Mandelstam, M. (1998). *An A-Z of community care law*. London: Jessica Kingsley Publishers.
McCarthy, M. (Ed.). (1989). *The new politics of welfare: An agenda for the 1990s* (pp. 22-52). London: Macmillan.

Meteyard, B. (1994). *Community care keyworker manual: A resource book for managers, practitioners and trainers* (2nd ed.). Brighton: Pavilion.

Ngan, R., & Wong, W. (1995). Injustice in family care of the Chinese elderly in Hong Kong. *Journal of Aging & Social Policy, 7*(2), 77-94.

Payne, M. (1986). *Social care in the community*. London: Macmillan.

Ramon, S. (1991). Principles and conceptual knowledge. In S. Ramon (Ed.), *Beyond community care: Normalisation and integration work* (pp. 6-34). London: Macmillan.

Sainsbury, S. (1995). Disabled people and the personal social services. In D. Gladstone (Ed.), *British social welfare: Past, present, and future* (pp.183-194). London: University College London Press.

Secretary of State for Health, Secretary of State for Social Security, Secretary of State for Wales, & Secretary of State for Scotland (DHSS, UK). (1989). *White Paper: Caring for People: Community care in the next decade and beyond*. London: HMSO. (Cmnd.849)

Segal, S. P. (1979). Community care and deinstitutionalization: A review. *Social Work, 24*(6), 521-527.

Tester, S. (1996). Women and community care. In C. Hallett (Ed.), *Women and social policy: An introduction* (pp. 132-145). London: Prentice Hall.

Titmuss, R. M. (1968). Community care: Fact or fiction? In *Commitment to welfare* (Chapter IX, pp. 104-109). London: George Allen and Unwin Ltd.

Walker, A. (1981). Community care and the elderly in Great Britain: Theory and practice. *International Journal of Health Services, 11*(4), 541-557.

Walker, A. (1982). The meaning and social division of community care. In A. Walker (Ed.), *Community care: The family, the state, and social policy* (pp. 13-39). Oxford: Basil Blackwell & Martin Robertson.

Walker, A. (1989). Community care. In M. McCarthy (Ed.), *The new politics of welfare: An agenda for the 1990s* (pp. 203-224). London: Macmillan.

Walker, A. (1997). Community care policy: From consensus to conflict. In J. Bornat, J. Johnson, C. Pereira, D. Pilgrim, & F. Williams (Eds.), *Community care: A reader* (2nd ed.) (pp. 196-220). London: The Open University.

Yeung, S. (1992). The community care policy of services for the elderly in Hong Kong: A critique. *Hong Kong Journal of Gerontology, 6*(2), 8-12.

<u>In Chinese (titles translated)</u>

Chang, Y. C., & Wang, S. (1999). Improving "Social Welfare Communitilization Study"–A case study in Kong-Shen of Koushung County. Sponsored by the Ministry of Interior, ROC Government. Taipei, February, 1999.

Chen, L. Y. (1995). Community care: Concepts and strategies, presented at the Conference of Community Care from Taiwan and Hong Kong, Taipei, July 1995.

Chen, M. L. (1995). The introduction of the "Community Care Promotion Committee." In M. L. Chen and others (Eds.), *The Handbook of the "Conference of Community Care in Taiwan"* (pp. 11-12). Taipei: Ministry of Interior and Social Affairs Department of Taipei Government.

Chen, W. S. (1997). Motivating "social welfare communitilization": Policy plan & operation. *Journal of Community Development, 77,* 7-12.

Chen, Y. J. (1998). The operational work on community care for the elderly: Concerns about the elderly who live alone. *Journal of Community Development, 83,* 244-257.

Chow, N. W. S. (1988). Family care and the limit of institutional care. *Hong Kong Journal of Gerontology, 2*(2), 25-27.

Fu, L. Y., Chou, Y. C., Houng, Y. T., & Chen, S. F. (2000). Life needs survey for persons with disabilities in Taipei City. Taipei: Taipei City Government.

Hu, Y. H. (1995). *Three generalizations: Myth and trap.* Taipei: Chu-lieu Publication Company.

Huang, G. B., & Chen, L. Y. (1996). Community care. In Kan, B. G. and others (Eds.), *Community work: Theory and practice* (pp. 327-357). Taipei: Wu-nan Publishing Company.

Kan, B. G. (1993). The application of community care: How to care for the aged in the community. In Z.Y. Gung & W. S. Ngan (Eds.), *Community Administration Work for Elderly Group* (pp. 165-184). Hong Kong: Chi-Shen Sir.

Kan, B. G. (1995). Community care: Concepts and principles of Implementation. *Journal of Community Development, 69,* 132-141.

Lee, G. S. (1987). The exploration and analysis of "Community care" policy.

Lee, S. C. (1993). Governmental housing services for the elderly in Hong Kong. *Hong Kong Journal of Gerontology, 7*(2), 37-52.

Leu, B. C. (1995). People attitudes and social welfare. In the National Association of Modern Welfare (Ed.), *Social welfare in Taiwan: Perspectives from non-governmental organizations* (pp. 67-102). Taipei: Wunan Publication Company.

Lou, S. H. (1996). Community work & community care. *Welfare Society, 54,* 9-13.

Lou, S. H. (1998). Community resources maintaining community care. *Journal of Community Development, 81,* 259-269.

Shieh, M. E. (1997). Based on the needs of community care for the disabled elderly exploring how to build services networks. *Journal of Sociology of the National Jenq-chu University, 27,* 47-88.

Shieh, M. E., & Lieu, S. G. (1996). Needs survey of community care for the disabled elderly. *Journal of Elderly Education, 8,* 51-60.

Shu, J. (1980). *Community and community development.* Taipei: Jenq-jong Books.

Shu, J. (1985). *Community development–Method and research.* Taipei: Chinese Culture University.

Su, G. H. (1995). The developmental directions of community care in Taiwan, presented at the Conference of Community Care from Taiwan and Hong Kong, Taipei, July 1995.

Su, G. H. (1994a). Community care model for the disabled people. *Journal of Community Development, 66,* 23-27.

Su, G. H. (1994b). Community care: Current situations and future development in Taiwan, Presented at the Conference on "Community Care and Chinese Community–Experiences Sharing between Main-land China, Taiwan, Macao, and Hong Kong," October 1994, pp. 55-62.

Su, G. H. (1996). *Community work: Theory and practice.* Taipei: Chu-lieu Publishing Company.

Su, G. H. (1998). Community care: Principles & methods. In the Community Empowering Society, ROC (Ed.), *Social welfare communitilization* (pp. 97-124). Taipei: Community Empowering Society, ROC.

Tung, S. B. (1971). *Community organization and community development.* Nantou, Taiwan: Taiwan Provincial Government.

Wang, C. C. (1990). Community social work–strategy for extending community care. In 1989/1990 "Community development in 1990s" (pp. 33-36). Hong Kong: Community Development Unit of Social Service United Association in Hong Kong.

Wang, F. (1998). The development of East Asia and social welfare: State, development strategy, and ideology, paper presented at the Conference on Social Welfare Development in Taiwan: Past, present, and future, Taiwan, April, 1998.

Won, W. D. (1998). The exploration of carrying out welfare communitilization. *Social Welfare Bio-monthly Journal, 135,* 38-45.

Young, S. Z. (1997). Practical operation of 'Welfare Communitilization.' *Journal of Community Development, 77,* 50-56.

Governmental Documents in Taiwan

1997 Protection Act of Persons with Disabilities. Taipei: ROC Government.

1997 the Elderly Welfare Act. Taipei: ROC Government.

Chang-hwa County Government. (1998). Fiscal budget plan on social welfare. Chang-hwa, Taiwan: Chang-hwa County Government.

Chang-hwa County Government. (1999). Fiscal budget plan on social welfare. Chang-hwa, Taiwan: Chang-hwa County Government.

Chang-hwa County Government. (1999-2000). Fiscal budget plan on social welfare. Chang-hwa, Taiwan: Chang-hwa County Government.

Department of Social Affairs, Ministry of Interior, R.O.C. (2000a). Welfare Subvention Regulations for Promoting Social Welfare. Taipei: Ministry of Interior, ROC Government.

Department of Social Affairs, Ministry of Interior, R.O.C. (2000b). Welfare Subvention Programs and Standards for Promoting Social Welfare. Taipei: Ministry of Interior, ROC Government.

Department of Social Affairs, Ministry of Interior (1994). The Principles of Social Welfare Policy and Programs. Worded by the Executive Yuan, R. O. C., July 1994. Taipei: Ministry of Interior, ROC Government.

Department of Social Affairs, Ministry of Interior (1996). Improving Social Welfare Communitilization: Directions of Implementation. Worded by the Social Affairs Department, Ministry of Interior, ROC. December 1996.

Ministry of Health of ROC. (1998). Three years of long-term care plan. Taipei: Ministry of Health, ROC Government.

Ministry of Interior of ROC. (1998). Fiscal budget plan on social welfare. Taipei: Ministry of Interior, ROC Government.

Ministry of Interior of ROC. (1999). Fiscal budget plan on social welfare. Taipei: Ministry of Interior, ROC Government.

Ministry of Interior of ROC. (1999-2000). Fiscal budget plan on social welfare. Taipei: Ministry of Interior, ROC Government.

Statistics Department, Ministry of Interior (1996). Survey Report of the disabled people in Taiwan. Taipei: Ministry of Interior, ROC Government.

Statistics Department, Ministry of Interior (2000). Survey Report of the disabled people in Taiwan. Taipei: Ministry of Interior, ROC Government.

Tainan City Government. (1998). Fiscal budget plan on social welfare. Tainan, Taiwan: Tainan City Government.

Tainan City Government. (1999). Fiscal budget plan on social welfare. Tainan, Taiwan: Tainan City Government.

Tainan City Government. (1999-2000). Fiscal budget plan on social welfare. Tainan, Taiwan: Tainan City Government.

Taipei City Government. (1994). White Paper of Taipei City Government. Taipei: Taipei City Government.

Taipei City Government. (1999). Introduction of the elderly welfare services in Taipei City. September, 1999. Taipei: Taipei City Government.

Taipei City Government. (1998). Fiscal budget plan on social welfare. Taipei: Taipei City Government.

Taipei City Government. (1999). Fiscal budget plan on social welfare. Taipei: Taipei City Government.

Taipei City Government. (1999-2000). Fiscal budget plan on social welfare. Taipei: Taipei City Government.

Yi-lan County Government. (1998). Fiscal budget plan on social welfare. Yi-lan, Taiwan: Yi-lan County Government.

Yi-lan County Government. (1999). Fiscal budget plan on social welfare. Yi-lan, Taiwan: Yi-lan County Government.

Yi-lan County Government. (1999-2000). Fiscal budget plan on social welfare. Yi-lan, Taiwan: Yi-lan County Government.

Governmental Documents in Hong Kong

Hong Kong Government. (1994). Report of the Working Group on Care of the Elderly. Hong Kong: Government Printers.

Hong Kong Government. (1994). Report of the Working Group on Care for the Elderly. Hong Kong: Government Printers. August 1994.

Hong Kong Government. (1991). Social welfare into the 1990s and Beyond–White Paper. Hong Kong: Government Printers.

Hong Kong Government. (1985). The Five Year Plan for Social Welfare Development in Hong Kong-Review 1985. Hong Kong: Government Printers.

Hong Kong Government. (1980). The Five Year Plan for Social Welfare Development in Hong Kong-Review 1980. Hong Kong: Government Printers.

Hong Kong Government. (1977). The Five Year Plan for Social Welfare Development in Hong Kong-Review 1977. Hong Kong: Government Printers.

Hong Kong Government. (1977). Green Paper "Services for the Elderly." Hong Kong: Government Printers. November 1977.

Hong Kong Government. (1965). White Paper "Aims and Policy for Social Welfare in Hong Kong." Hong Kong: Government Printers.

The Efficacy of Involuntary Treatment in the Community: Consumer and Service Provider Perspectives

Lisa Brophy
David Ring

SUMMARY. Since the passing of the Mental Health Act (1986), Victoria, Australia, has implemented Community Treatment Orders (CTOs) as an alternative to involuntary inpatient admission for patients who are assessed as unable to be treated less restrictively but in an effort to avoid frequent hospital admissions. It is estimated that currently 3,000 people are annually placed on CTOs in this Australian state. The following article will review existing international and national literature on the subject of forms of involuntary treatment in the community before reporting on the findings of a research project that focused on gaining both consumer and service provider perspectives on the efficacy of CTOs. The

Lisa Brophy, BBSC, BSW, is Master of Policy and Law (LaTrobe University) Adjunct Lecturer in the School of Social Work and Social Policy, La Trobe University, Chief Social Worker, North West Area Mental Health Service, and Chairperson, The Mental Health Legal Centre (E-mail address: Lisa.Brophy@mh.org.au). David Ring, BA Monash, BSW (Hons) is affiliated with the Melbourne University, Mental Health Legal Centre Inc. (Victoria) Policy Worker (E-mail: David_Ring@fcl.fl.asn.au).

Special thanks are extended to Dr. Jim Campbell (Queens University, Belfast) for his assistance with the revision and Associate Professor Bill Healy (LaTrobe University) for his valued input into earlier drafts.

[Haworth co-indexing entry note]: "The Efficacy of Involuntary Treatment in the Community: Consumer and Service Provider Perspectives." Brophy, Lisa, and David Ring. Co-published simultaneously in *Social Work in Mental Health* (The Haworth Social Work Practice Press, an imprint of The Haworth Press, Inc.) Vol. 2, No. 2/3, 2004, pp. 157-174; and: *Social Work Approaches in Health and Mental Health from Around the Globe* (ed: Metteri et al.) The Haworth Social Work Practice Press, an imprint of The Haworth Press, Inc., 2004, pp. 157-174. Single or multiple copies of this article are available for a fee from The Haworth Document Delivery Service [1-800-HAWORTH, 9:00 a.m. - 5:00 p.m. (EST). E-mail address: docdelivery@haworthpress.com].

research method was largely qualitative, involving three focus groups attended by 30 consumers, as well as 18 individual interviews with service providers. The aim of the project was to offer a voice to both consumers and service providers about their experiences and views of current practice and policy implementation in an area that can have a profound effect on the rights of consumers. Findings suggest that CTOs involve complex decision-making that tests professionals' ability to make judgements about legal and clinical processes. Consumers were generally dissatisfied with many aspects of the use of CTOs and both groups tended to view CTOs as stigmatising and disempowering. There were a variety of views expressed about the process of admission, discharge, and community supports. The article concludes by discussing the findings in the context of existing national and international literature and makes a number of recommendations about law reform, and service provision. *[Article copies available for a fee from The Haworth Document Delivery Service: 1-800-HAWORTH. E-mail address: <docdelivery@haworthpress.com> Website: <http://www.HaworthPress.com> © 2004 by The Haworth Press, Inc. All rights reserved.]*

KEYWORDS. Involuntary treatment, outpatient commitment, consumer perspectives, mental health law, community treatment orders (CTOs)

INTRODUCTION

In the last decades of the twentieth century, policy makers in many developed countries have sought to find ways of closing large psychiatric institutions and caring for and treating people with mental health problems (Scull, 1988). It has become increasingly apparent that more coercive approaches have been used, not just to prevent relapse, but also to manage risk.

For example, in the UK a number of authors have highlighted a policy context in which the rights of clients are often compromised by the competing demands of professional power, community rejection, and resource limitations (Bartlett & Wright, 1999; Bean, 2001). Although there is no history of the use of community treatment orders (CTOs) in this part of the world, the current reform of the Mental Health Act (England and Wales), 1983 suggests that such mechanisms may well be in place in a few years time, despite the misgivings of some professional opinion (Brown, 2002). On the other hand, in New Zealand, psychiatrists have reported some limited success in using CTOs, particularly with high risk groups (Dawson & Romans, 2001).

In North America, where most states use compulsory treatment, a number of studies have focused on the impact of such policies. Calsyn, Winter, and Morse (2000) found that, when comparing compliance to treatment between those mandated and those non-mandated consumers, there was no clear indicator to suggest any difference in health outcomes after 12 months. Welxer and Winck (1998) found that health workers became more 'police like,' at the expense of a therapeutic role, when using such legislation. Hiday and Scheid-Cook (1991) have pointed out a less restrictive position for workers in some U.S. states because an outpatient commitment does not allow for compulsory medication (or this is discouraged practice), and consumers are not re-admitted to hospital for non-compliance alone. They describe the use of an assertive outreach model with mandatory powers (such as the propensity to make a person attend a consultation with psychiatric trained staff) rather than a method of treatment that involves compliance through the threat of hospitalisation or enforced treatment, such as medication.[1] Hiday and Scheid-Cook (1991) found that, with assertive outreach methods of compulsory follow-up, clinicians were often successful in gaining consumer co-operation with treatment. Stein and Test (1980) have also highlighted positive outcomes for assertive outreach in community mental health care and treatment. These studies may suggest that a reliance on involuntary treatment prevents more creative and attractive (for many consumers) treatment strategies. There is also a possible risk of an erosion of service provider skills and use of therapeutic approaches if professionals are over-committed to compulsory methods of intervention.

The Australian Context–Community Treatment Orders (CTOs)

This international context is important in understanding the development and use of CTOs in Australia generally, and more particularly Victoria. Victoria operates within a federal Australian system of six states and two territories, each of which has responsibility for their own mental health law. As a consequence, each state varies to some degree in terms of the treatment and care of people who receive mental health services. In the 1980s in Victoria the then Labor government introduced a raft of progressive legislation for people with disabilities as part of a social justice strategy; this included, for example, legislation on intellectual disability and guardianship. The Mental Health Act of 1986 differed, however, because, like much legislative reform occurring throughout the world at the time, it tried to achieve a balance between individual rights and the rights of wider society when considering treatment and care in the community. Factors created by an ongoing process of deinstitutionalisation led in 1988 to an amendment of the Mental Health Act to allow for the use of CTOs. The Act defines the concept as follows:

> "Community Treatment Order" means an order requiring treatment for mental illness of a person who is at large in the community but does not apply to a person in prison or a patient in an approved mental health service. (Mental Health Act of 1986 (s.3 def))

CTOs were considered to be a logical consequence of deinstitutionalisation because they reinforced the notion that mental health care, even involuntary treatment, should as far as possible be located in the community. Despite the humanitarian ethos which appears to underpin such shifts from hospital to community based treatment, CTOs imply considerable state power over the lives of the individuals involved; for example, consumers[2] who have their CTO revoked may be apprehended by the police (s.14 (4A) (b)). Although CTOs were initially designed to facilitate the discharge of inpatients into the community and to subsequently have their CTO monitored by outpatient clinics, subsequent amendments have made it possible to place consumers directly onto a CTO, the so-called 'lounge chair' admission. As a result of such practices CTOs began to act as a direct substitute for involuntary admission as an inpatient. It was not until amendments in 1996 (Department of Health & Community Services, 1995) that separate criteria were created and defined under the Act. In Victoria a person must now meet all five criteria of Section 14 (1A) of the Mental Health Act of 1986 to be placed on a community treatment order. The criteria are:

a. the person appears to be mentally ill; and
b. the person's mental illness requires immediate treatment can be obtained by making the person subject to a community treatment order; and
c. because of a person's mental illness, the person should be made subject to a community treatment order for his or her health or safety (whether to prevent a deterioration in the person's physical or mental condition or otherwise) or for the protection of members of the public; and
d. the person has refused treatment or is unable to consent to the necessary treatment for the mental illness; and
e. the person cannot receive adequate treatment for the mental illness in a manner less restrictive of that person's freedom of decision and action.

An authorised psychiatrist makes the Order (s.14 (1)) and the authorised psychiatrist or their delegate is then required to monitor the treatment (s.14

(2)(a)). The number of the times the Order can be extended is indefinite (s.14 (7)) and an Order may be revoked if the authorised psychiatrist is reasonably satisfied that the person failed to comply (s.14 (4)(b)). This person would be returned to an inpatient facility (s.14 (4A)).

A person must have their Order reviewed by the Mental Health Review Board (MHRB), an external review tribunal made up of community, legal and psychiatrist members, within an 8-week period and thereafter at intervals not exceeding 12 months (s30 (1)(a)). The person may appeal to the MHRB at any time, requiring the Board to commence the hearing of an appeal without delay (s.29 (4)). In Victoria, the authorised psychiatrist–not the Board–makes the Order. The Victorian legislation does not outline what the treatment should be. Therefore the Board can make no decision with regard to a person's actual treatment, only that they receive treatment (Lee, 1993).

CTOs have increasingly become part of the landscape of psychiatric services in Victoria, Australia. It is estimated that around 3,000 Orders were made in the year 1999[3] and many of these people have had their orders extended on numerous times. It was suggested not long after CTOs were introduced that they were likely to become an increasingly familiar feature of psychiatric services (Lee, 1993) and indeed it appears that they are being increasingly relied upon to ensure continuity of care. Furthermore, it is likely that many people will remain on CTOs for long periods when reviews are held only annually.

Various factors may be seen to be the driving forces behind the increased use of CTOs both in Australia and internationally. They may be improving the efficiency of service delivery by enabling less emphasis on, usually very expensive, inpatient care, and in doing so, support the commitment to treat people in the least restrictive environment possible (Health & Community Services: Victorian Mental Health Services: The Framework for Service Delivery: 1996). These orders also set up mechanisms that assist in ensuring that people discharged from inpatient services are offered treatment in the community (Lee, 1993). This relates also to the importance in mental health services currently being placed on managing issues of potential risk, such as the possibility that the person may harm themselves or others (Rose, 1998). Other driving forces include research that suggests that CTOs may offer significant benefits to consumers compared with involuntary inpatient admissions or no treatment at all. Although this research is not uncontested there are examples of studies that have found significant benefits for patients in relation to a range of factors including reduced rates of hospital admission, improved insight, better relationships with carers, greater connection to support and treatment services, and increased protection against harm to self or others (Dedman, 1991; Carne, 1991; Turner, 1994; Freckelton, 1998; McIvor, 1998; Muirhead, 2000).

However, people on CTOs in Victoria may be seen to be particularly disadvantaged in a number of different ways beyond the obvious issue of being coerced into treatment. For example, it has been argued that many people on CTOs may have limited awareness of their rights and many people, especially those in rural communities, have limited access to specialised legal services (MHLC Annual Report, 2000). It has also been suggested that CTOs can be poorly administered (*Wilson v Mental Health Review Board and others* [2000] VSC 404 (6 October)) and that services lack the resources required to ensure accountability and fully appreciate the responsibilities that CTOs represent. There is also some concern, consistent with what has been previously mentioned, that, at practice level, the more traditional skills of staff in engaging clients, or helping consumers to achieve some kind of insight, may be lost or eroded by this more coercive policy environment (Ring, Brophy, & Gimlinger, 2001).

CTOs– "The Lived Experience"

Despite the fact that the use of CTOs has become more commonplace in Victoria since they were introduced in 1988, there has been limited research, especially in relation to consumer perspectives (McDonnell & Bartholomew, 1997). McDonnell and Bartholomew (1997) comment that research that has been undertaken tends to focus on "treatment compliance and readmission rates as primary indicators of success" (p. 27), rather than focussing on the expressed needs and views of patients.

External reviews of the lawful implementation of involuntary treatment in the community are carried out through administrative review processes that apply to all jurisdictions in Australia, but there is limited automatic review by the Mental Health Review Board (or the equivalent), even though people can appeal at any time against their orders (Cook, 2000; Model Mental Health Legislation, 1995). Although not comprehensively researched, there is evidence to support the contention that the external review process may encourage what Brophy (1995) has described as an 'informal discharge rate,' that is a high proportion of discharges occurring just prior to the scheduled date of review (O'Reilly, Komer, & Dunbar, 1999; MHRB, 2000). Victoria has one of the longest periods before compulsory review; therefore, this pattern of discharge is of particular significance in terms of clients' rights. Lee (1993) has argued that such waiting "may engender feelings of hopelessness and loss of control over their [consumers] lives" (p. 28).

In terms of future research into the impact and effectiveness of CTOs for consumers of mental health services, it can be argued that descriptive, quantitative approaches focused largely on rates of readmission, compliance, and fiscally derived concerns may not be totally adequate in assessing the overall efficacy of CTOs (McDonnell & Bartholomew, 1997). Complex issues of care and control (*parens patriae*) and social justice (Moore, Beazley, & Maelzer, 1998) also implies the need to address the 'lived experience' of those involved in involuntary community treatment, including consumers as well as professionals. This is the approach taken in this article.

METHOD

The following study used a mixed method approach to ascertain consumer and professional views about the operation of CTOs in Victoria. Although some quantitative data was collected, for example demographic characteristics of participants and Likert-type responses elicited from professionals to test their levels of knowledge and satisfaction with CTOs, the study used a generally qualitative approach. Qualitative methodology is the choice when seeking meaning from human experiences which are sometimes difficult to capture using, for example, survey techniques (Miller & Dingwall, 1997). The researchers viewed this as an important approach to examine how both consumers and practitioners viewed how involuntary community treatment processes operated in the state of Victoria, Australia.

Sampling

The investigators conducted focus groups with 30 consumers recruited from three diverse areas: rural Victoria, outer southeast Melbourne, and inner north Melbourne. Interviews were also carried out with 18 service providers randomly selected via telephone request from a range of psychiatric services. These included social workers, occupational therapists, consumer advocates welfare workers, psychiatrists, psychiatric nurses, solicitors, and medical records clerks. These people were employed in the following service types: psychiatric disability support services, community health centres, the Department of Human Services, and area mental health services, which included crisis assessment teams, continuing care teams, and community care units.

Study Instruments

Two instruments were used to capture the views of respondents. The first was applied to the sample of consumers to help explore their understanding and attitudes to CTOs, as they had been operationalised in Victoria. A number of open-ended questions were asked around eight key themes: what the purpose of CTOs were; why they were needed; whether there were any benefits; whether there were any problems; what respondents knew about the discharge process; whether CTOs could be improved; life without a CTO; what treatments CTOs brought. The second instrument was designed to elucidate practice knowledge about the use of CTOs by professionals. A mixture of Likert-type and open-ended responses were used to explore the following themes: overall professional and client satisfaction with CTOs; whether CTOs were empowering and helped in developing consumer insight; knowledge about how the law prescribed conditions for treatment and discharge; perceptions about the efficacy of CTOs; and the strengths and weaknesses of CTOs.

Research Process

The research took place over a four-month period in 2000, with the assistance of a social work student on placement[4] at the Mental Health Legal Centre Inc.[5] The 30 consumers were interviewed in three focus groups. It has been argued that focus groups are considered to be the most appropriate method for engaging consumers in discussions about their experience of involuntary treatment in the community (Moore, Beazley, & Maelzer, 1998). During these groups two facilitators were used in exploring responses to questions whilst another person recorded the data. One of the facilitators was also a consumer of psychiatric services, and it was anticipated that this would assist in creating a non-threatening and potentially emancipatory environment in the focus groups (Moore, Beazley, & Maelzer, 1998). Individual interviews were carried out with professionals by the same person, thus ensuring a sense of continuity and evenness of process with each of the respondents.

Data Analysis

After schedules were completed the researchers summarised and examined the data, in the process identifying themes that had emerged in the research process. Although this is necessarily an inexact, interpretive procedure, a degree of consistency was introduced through the use of cross checking of responses between the two researchers to establish meaning and priority of responses. Both authors have long-standing knowledge and experience of the use of CTOs in Victoria.

FINDINGS

Background Data

The focus group participants were most likely to be male, in their early 40s, have a diagnosis of schizophrenia and be living on state benefit. The majority of respondents' education level was of secondary school standard, with most people living alone or in supported accommodation. Most focus group participants were currently in receipt of a CTO, sometimes for long periods. For example, one participant in this group described being on a CTO for 6 years, another was still on a CTO after 4 years. Another estimated that he had been on a CTO '3 times.'

Six social workers, and two of each of the following professional groups participated–medical officers/psychiatrists, occupational therapists, lawyers, psychiatric nurses. In addition one medical records officer, an advocate and a welfare worker were included. Most of the sample was women and all had a wide experience of working in the mental health field.

Consumers' Views

When the data were collected, three main themes emerged from the group interviews with consumers.

Understanding the Purpose of CTOs

Most consumers expressed a general view that CTOs had functional purposes, for example, to ensure further treatment at a time of crisis, or as one respondent put it, it might, "get you into hospital without the red tape." These participants talked about feeling safer and more secure while on a CTO, knowing that services may be more responsive. Many of the participants acknowledged that there were times when they, or other people they knew, became very unwell, usually associated with not complying with treatment, and they believed that involuntary treatment, either in the form of inpatient admission or a CTO, was appropriate to deal with this crisis. Some consumers believed that they were put on a CTO because they had been violent to other people; one specifically mentioned that this had occurred while he was in a psychiatric inpatient unit. Perhaps for such reasons some consumers felt that CTOs could prevent violence carried out against family members or members of the public. On the other hand, there was a concern amongst many that these Orders were punitive, for example, one consumer compared them to a "CBO," [6] another thought it was the equivalent of "being in jail without any walls." The underlying threat of sanctions associated with CTOs was also commonly cited. As one respondent put it, "if you did not take drugs then the police would come and take you to hospital." A sense of anger about these threats emerged in the group interviews; one respondent thought he had been placed on a CTO "because they're [professionals] *fascists.*"

Somewhat worryingly, most of the participants did not seem to have any consistent understanding of criteria associated with CTOs, for example no one was aware of the specific five conditions outlined in the legislation. The overall impression that emerged was that consumers assumed that this was a simple decision made by their treating doctor, somehow divorced from law and regulation.

The Strengths and Weaknesses of CTOs

Consumers expressed a number of concerns about the negative impact of CTOs on their lives. For example one group respondent felt that the label associated with the Order was more stigmatising than having the diagnosis of mental illness. This theme was highlighted by another consumer who felt insecure about their position at work and was worried that their employer would find out they had been on a CTO. A constant theme that emerged in the group interviews was the intense dislike of the forced nature of treatment, particularly the use of injections to ensure compliance. An argument was made by many group participants, echoing the views of service users elsewhere in the world (Read & Reynolds, 1996), that they would prefer a range of other therapeutic responses, apart from the use of medication, and be able to have "someone who would really listen." Most consumers reported receiving only medication from the Area Mental Health Services, although four participants were able to identify other forms of help which they had received including–a referral to other allied health services, psychological and 'talking treatments,' and use of alternative therapies.

This sense that professionals were not responsive enough to consumers' needs was reinforced in the views of a respondent who complained that his doctor was only available in normal working hours, this was problematic because of their own nine-to-five work commitments. What were needed, it was argued, were properly funded out-of-hour services. Many consumers highlighted the often punitive, restrictive nature of CTOs, although one woman felt that it helped her to comply with her medication and deal with the associated fear of losing her mind if she stopped taking medication.

Apart from these individualised views, most respondents could not identify any ways in which CTOs could be improved, perhaps because of generalised feelings of powerlessness and a belief that they did not, and could not, have any valid input into the decision-making processes involving such Orders.

Knowledge About Discharge Procedures

Although consumers did not generally understand the five involuntary admission criteria, they seemed to be aware of the need to become involved with the mental health services in a range of ways, to enable this to happen. For example, one consumer stated that *"you had to dress up well and play the game and stay in the good books of the doctor,"* and another explained, *"you need to let the CATT [7] team come and speak to you."* Many seemed to recognise the need to ask to receive and comply with treatment from their doctor. One consumer knew that the Mental Health Review Board could become involved in the discharge, but in their case was pessimistic that this would work for them. Some consumers made a number of recommendations about how the system could be improved. For example, it was suggested that the length of time before a Review should be shortened to, say, every 6 months. Another respondent felt that the service providers should be more efficient in their planning and resourcing of Boards so that consumers would have a fairer chance of discharge. A focus group member felt that the criteria for involuntary treatment were too rigid and should be made more flexible to enhance the rights of consumers. It was of some surprise, given these negative responses, that only one person stated that CTOs should be removed totally from the mental health legislation.

Professionals' Views

When the data were collected, a number of themes emerged and are described in the next section.

The Function of CTOs and Their Impact on Consumers

It was clear from the consumer group interviews that many respondents were concerned and dissatisfied with the way CTOs had been used. Professional respondents, however, expressed more positive views about the operationalisation of the Orders.[8] Thirteen were either moderately satisfied with or very satisfied with the way Orders were used. For example one social worker felt that it *"provides a structure to the clinician's role,"* and a psychiatrist thought that it was a useful mechanism because it *"provides assertive outreach for clinicians."* On the other hand, most respondents seemed to recognise the potentially negative, stigmatising impact on consumers. Half of the sample thought that consumers were either moderately or very dissatisfied with CTOs. As one occupational therapist put it, *"Involuntary status makes them* [consumers] *feel as though they are still patients . . . leads to a loss of control over life."* Another respondent said *"it saves clinicians having to negotiate with consumers."* Only three professionals, two doctors and one occupational therapist, thought that CTOs had been an empowering experience for consumers. Reasons given for this response were generally focused on the positive lifestyle benefits, which flowed from appropriate use of medication. Other professionals in the sample tended to have more negative views around the coercive, restrictive effect Orders had for consumers.

Knowledge About How the Law Prescribed Conditions for Treatment and Discharge

Professionals were generally quite knowledgeable about the basic principles involved in the review procedure, although there was some divergence of opinion about what criteria would be used to judge whether a CTO should cease or continue. Compliance ($n = 12$) was the most commonly stated reason for discharge, followed next by insight ($n = 9$). For example, one psychiatrist made judgements based on the consumers *"Engagement with treatment . . . acceptance of a mental illness and compliance."* A stable mental state and the notion of 'engagement with service' were less frequently mentioned. In relation to why a CTO might be justified in the first instance, only four respondents identified the need to meet the five legislative criteria, and four said that a forthcoming MHRB would be factors in the discharge process, as one nurse put it, *"so they don't have present before the MHRB–it is a time factor."* When asked about how long, on average, consumers had been placed on CTOs by their service, eleven said over one year. This may reflect the relatively long period of CTO application before a review is necessary, when compared to other Australian states. The literature on the use of CTOs suggests that practitioners face many competing ethical and clinical demands in making judgements in this complex area of work. For this reason the researchers sought to explore the possible tension between 'best interest practice' and 'strict adherence to the legislation.' Only three of the people interviewed believed that strict adherence to the legislation was more important–*"the Act is more important than best practice"* (social worker), whereas eight favoured best interest practice– *"If a person relapses this reflects negatively on professional practice"* (psychiatric nurse). The others took a hybrid position, for example a lawyer highlighted the ambiguity of decision making in the following way: "Best interest can be interpreted paternally, oppressively, or rights-based legislation can be misinterpreted."

Perceptions About the Efficacy of CTOs

Literature on the subject suggests that the complicated legal, social, and professional factors involved in the use and administration of CTOs makes it difficult to ascertain efficacy. The researcher sought to use a number of questions to test respondents' ideas on this concept. For example, they were asked, in terms of their experience and judgement, whether clients in receipt of a CTO would relapse clinically more frequently than those not on a CTO. There was no consensus in the group on this matter, with views evenly spread across professional groupings. When asked about how much input consumers had in the operationalisation of their CTO, again there were a variety of responses, but over half thought there was usually little or none. As one social worker explained, *"Patients have very little input, it's a medical decision."* When asked to compare this form of consumer involvement alongside work with clients who had voluntary status, ten respondents thought that they would be treated differently. As another social worker stated, the *"Voluntary patient is able to negotiate more* [there] *is a greater degree of equality."* In contrast, and perhaps reflecting the contemporary debate within mental health policy about the right to treatment, one respondent felt that, *"You would expect that a person who is involuntary would have less* (input into treatment), *however, due to the nature of the illness and team support, they sometimes have more."*

Given the many negative perceptions that consumers have about their experiences of CTOs, it was felt important to ask professionals to judge advantages and disadvantages associated with this process. Rank ordered, beginning with the most frequently identified problems, they were as follows: lack of control over life; loss of freedom; too restrictive; lack of choice about treatment; disempowering experience; stigmatising; reduction in life opportunities. A number of advantages were, however, acknowledged, particularly the opportunity for an improvement in mental health and access to treatment. Other factors included access to a case manager and, as result, resources. Despite this optimism, over half of the respondents felt that CTOs may not always help people become connected with other services. This may be because there is no statutory requirement to provide such services; these are often contingent upon the activity of the case manager.

Finally, when asked about how CTOs could be improved, the professional group made a number of suggestions. A wide variety of responses were made, including the need to improve the administration of CTOs, a greater need to involve the consumer's family and wider community, increase psycho education and a shorter review period.

DISCUSSION OF FINDINGS

This study sought to use a triangulated approach to capture consumer and service provider perceptions of CTOs. A number of themes emerged from the research which are of note and which may have relevance for such settings in other parts of the world. This is an important area of study because of the complex interface between legal and clinical matters, which makes professional judgement difficult and involves considerable restrictions on the rights of citizens (McIvor, 1998).

Perhaps CTOs are likely to be favoured by the general community, in that they represent one way of ensuring that people deinstitutionalised from psychiatric hospitals remain connected with treatment or because of the fears about the presence of mental health service consumers within the general community. This research seeks to contribute to an emerging discourse that raises important social justice and human rights issues and challenging questions worthy of broader public debate (McIvor, 1998). We cannot risk confining decisions regarding the ongoing control of fellow citizens who have historically been marginalised because of their otherness. This is a particularly important issue at a time when, decision making by professionals takes place in a generally poorly resourced and increasingly defensive practice environment. The capacity of professionals to make such difficult judgements has already been convincingly questioned in the context of institutionalisation (Rosenhan, 1973) and it may be that community based treatment will not remain immune to such challenges.

It was apparent from the findings that consumers are particularly unsure about legal processes and their rights within the legislation, an issue which has been raised by researchers in the context of mental health law in the UK (Campbell et al., 2001; Hatfield & Antcliff, 2001). For example, consumers indicated that they did not understand the five involuntary admission criteria or the necessity that they be met before involuntary detention can be made; this is despite direct reference in the Mental Health Act of 1986 (Vic) to the importance of patients having the right to information (s.18). Perhaps more surprisingly the majority of service providers did not highlight the importance of the five criteria in their discussion of why people are discharged from CTOs. They, like the consumers, tended to refer indirectly to the criteria through their discussion of the issues of compliance and being seen to have 'insight.' It is of interest to note that, while consumers could not articulate that the mental health service had to prove that a person met the five criteria to place them on a CTO, they had shared understandings about how to improve the chances of being discharged. The service provider responses tended to locate insight with compliance with medication, and this formed the primary basis to any decision about discharge.

The responses suggest that consumers may see CTOs as a method of 'fast tracking' themselves into hospital if required in a crisis, or perhaps gaining access to resources. In a similar way, some professionals in the survey felt that this may be a beneficial effect of the CTO, although there was an acknowledgment that this issue of access to resources was not fully embedded in the legislation and was contingent upon the activity of the case manager.

One common area of agreement between the two groups was the concern that CTOs had the propensity to be stigmatising and disempowering. There were also some concerns, particularly amongst consumers, about the way CTOs were administered, for example, in terms of what factors are involved in deciding about discharge and whether the length of time consumers have to wait for reviews is too long. There was also a general concern about the emphasis placed on medication as the primary, and sometimes only, treatment offered.

CONCLUSION

In conclusion it is important to recognise that the use of CTOs may be used appropriately as an alternative to assertive outpatient treatment and support. However, as stated above, CTOs impact on issues of social justice and human rights. The experience in Victoria is particularly significant in that CTOs have been implemented for many years and what is described here are only some of the many factors that appear to influence the use of CTOs in Victoria. Even so, CTOs, in one form or another, are rapidly becoming a feature of mental health legislation worldwide. This is despite the lack of strong evidence for their effectiveness and broad based community support. The findings of this study suggest that there is more work to be done to ensure that consumers are enabled to become more knowledgeable about their legal rights and views about how they are cared for and treated. It was apparent that there was a range of quite diverse opinions within the professional respondent group, which suggests that many aspects of the law and practice of CTOs may be contested, and in need of clarification, particularly about admission, discharge, and clinical interpretation. These issues are made that much more difficult if adequate community based resources are not made available to both consumers and professionals. The results of the above study suggest significant room for improvement in both development and implementation to ensure that CTOs reflect in practice the principles on which they are based.

NOTES

1. The Bazelon Center for Mental Health Law has summarised USA state statutes on involuntary outpatient commitment at http://www.webcom.com/bazelon/iocchart. html (date accessed 12/05/01).

2. This article uses the term consumers to describe people using psychiatric services or subject to community treatment orders.

3. Mental Health Review Board, Annual Report 2000-3000 individuals and 13,196 cases listed for a pop. of 3,500,000.

4. The authors would like to acknowledge Amanda Gimlinger, a Social Work Student at LaTrobe University for her work and assistance in undertaking this research.

5. The views expressed in this paper are those of the writers as social workers with an interest in this topic and do not express any endorsed policy position of the Mental Health Legal Centre Inc.

6. CBO–a Community Based Order issued within the criminal justice system.

7. Crisis Assessment and Treatment Team.

8. Some of the findings from the service provider interviews have been previously published in Ring, Brophy, and Gimlinger (2001) Examining Community Treatment Orders: A Preliminary Inquiry into their efficacy. *Health Issues*, March, 13-17.

REFERENCES

Bartlett, P. & Wright, D. (1999) Outside the Walls of the Asylum, London: Athlone.

Bazelon Centre for Mental Health Law, http;//www.bazelon.org/opcstud.html (revised March 16, 2001) Date of access: 12/05/01.

Bean, P. (2001) Mental Disorder and the Community, London: Palgrave.

Brophy, L. (1995) The impact of the Mental Health Review Board on Psychiatric services in Victoria. Unpublished master's thesis. La Trobe University.

Brown, D. (2002) Draft Mental Health Bill Receives Frosty Reception from Professionals, Community Care, 4/5/02. 18-19.

Calsyn, R., Winter, J. & Morse, G. (2000) Do Consumers who have a choice have better outcomes. *Community Mental Health Journal.* 36(3), 149-160.

Campbell, J., Brittan, F., Hamilton, B., Hughes, P., Manktelow, R. & Wilson, G. (2001) The Management and Supervision of Approved Social Workers: Aspects of Law Policy and Practice, *The Journal of Social Welfare and Family Law.*

Carne, J. (1991) A study of the effect and outcome of the use of community treatment orders and community counselling orders in New South Wales in 1991. Central Sydney Health Service, Sydney, Australia. Unpublished paper.

Cook, S. (2000) Relative CTO rights research project: Review of Australian legislative provisions. Prepared for the Mental Health Legal Centre Inc. Victoria. Unpublished paper.

Dawson, J. & Romans, S. (2001) Uses of CTOs in New Zealand: Early Findings, *Australian and New Zealand Journal of Psychiatry*, 35 : 190-195.

Dedman, P. (1990) Community treatment orders in Victoria, Australia. *Psychiatric Bulletin.* 14, 462-464.

Department of Health and Community Services (1996) Victorian Mental Health Services, The Proposed Framework for Service Delivery, Better Outcomes Through

Area Mental Health Services, Psychiatric Service Division, Victorian Government Department of Health.

Department of Health and Community Services (1995) Victorian Mental Health Services, Proposed Amendments to the Mental Health Act 1986, Psychiatric Service Division, Victorian Government Department of Health.

Freckleton (1998) Decision making about involuntary psychiatric treatment: An analysis of the principles behind Victorian practice. *Psychiatry, Psychology, and the Law.* 5(20), 249-264.

Hatfield, B. & Antcliff, V. (2001) Detention under the mental health act; balancing rights, risks and needs for services. *Journal of Social Welfare and Family Law,* 23, 2: 135-153.

Hiday, V.A. & Scheid-Cook, T.L (1991) Outpatient commitment for 'revolving door' patient 'compliance and treatment.' *Journal of Nervous and Mental Disease.* 179 (2), 83-88.

Lee, J. (1993) Community treatment orders: The Victorian experience. *Health Issues.* 34, 25-28.

McDonnell, E. & Bartholomew, T. (1997) Community treatment orders in Victoria: Emergent issues and anomalies. *Psychiatry, Psychology, and Law.* 4(1): 25-36.

McIvor, R. (1998) The community treatment order: Clinical and ethical issues. *Australian and New Zealand Journal of Psychiatry.* 32, 223-228.

Mental Health Act of 1986 (Vic).

Mental Health Act of 1996 (WA).

Mental Health Legal Centre (2000) *Annual Report 2000,* Mental Health Legal Centre, Victoria.

Mental Health Review Board Annual Report, 2000, *Annual Report 2000,* Mental Health Review Board, Victoria.

Miller, G. and Dingwall, R. (1997). *Context and Method in Qualitative Research.* London: Sage.

Model Mental Health Legislation (1995) Report to the Australian Health Ministers Advisory Council Working Group on Mental Health, Australian Health Ministers Advisory Council, Mental Health Branch, Canberra, ACT.

Moore, M., Beazley, S. & Maelzer, J. (1998) Research in Disability Issues. Buckingham: Open University Press.

Muirhead, D. (2000) Involuntary treatment of schizophrenia in the community; clinical effectiveness of community treatment orders with oral or depot medication in Victoria, Unpublished dissertation for section 11 examination, Royal Australian and New Zealand College of Psychiatrists.

O'Reilly, R., Komer, W. & Dunbar, S. (1999) Why are patients discharged by review boards? *Canadian Journal of Psychiatry.* 44, 259-263.

Ring, D., Brophy, L. & Gimlinger, A. (2001) Examining community treatment orders: A preliminary enquiry into their efficacy. *Health Issues.* 66 (March), 13-17.

Rose, N. (1998) Governing risky individuals: The role of psychiatry in new regimes of control. *Psychiatry, Psychology and the Law.* 5(2), 177-195.

Rosenhan, D. (1973) On being sane in insane places. *Science,* 179, 250-258.

Scull, A. (1977) Decarceration: community treatment and the deviant–A radical view. Englewood Cliffs. NY: Prentice Hall.

Stein, L.I. & Test, M.A. (1980) An alternative to mental hospital treatment: Conceptual model, treatment program and clinical evaluation. *Archives of General Psychiatry.* 37(4), 392-397.

The Herald Sun, 18th May, 2000, p. 10.

Turner, T. (1994) Compulsory treatment in the community: Some debating issues. *Psychiatric Bulletin.* 18(11), 657-659.

Welxer, D. & Winick, B. (1991) Essays in Therapeutic Jurisprudence. Durham, N.C., and U.S.A: Carolina Academic Press.

Wilson v Mental Health Review Board and others (2000) VSC 404 (6 October).

HIV/AIDS and Home Based Care in Botswana: Panacea or Perfidy?

Gloria Jacques
Christine Stegling

SUMMARY. The extent of the AIDS pandemic in Africa (and specifically in Botswana), and the lack of institutional frameworks to address concomitant issues, have necessitated the adoption of home based care for sufferers as national policy. The practice is beset by problems, given the severe symptomatic nature of the disease and the general lack of human and material resources to address the needs of patients and care-givers.

A study of one such programme in the Kweneng District of Botswana highlighted gender imbalances, poverty, lack of appropriate skills, over-involvement of the elderly, deficient specialised facilities, need for volunteer capacity building, inadequate income generating activities, insufficient counseling services, and culturally determined cognitive processes as areas requiring urgent attention. It is apparent that the programme needs strengthening through appropriate support mechanisms and that alternative strategies should be devised for those whose circumstances demand them.

Gloria Jacques is Senior Lecturer, Department of Social Work, University of Botswana, Private Bag 0022, Gaborone, Botswana (Email: jacques@mopipi.ub.bw). Christine Stegling is Director, Botswana Network on Ethics, Law, and HIV/AIDS (BONELA), P.O. Box 402958, Gaborone, Botswana (E-mail: bonela@botsnet.bw).

[Haworth co-indexing entry note]: "HIV/AIDS and Home Based Care in Botswana: Panacea or Perfidy?" Jacques, Gloria, and Christine Stegling. Co-published simultaneously in *Social Work in Mental Health* (The Haworth Social Work Practice Press, an imprint of The Haworth Press, Inc.) Vol. 2, No. 2/3, 2004, pp. 175-193; and: *Social Work Approaches in Health and Mental Health from Around the Globe* (ed: Metteri et al.) The Haworth Social Work Practice Press, an imprint of The Haworth Press, Inc., 2004, pp. 175-193. Single or multiple copies of this article are available for a fee from The Haworth Document Delivery Service [1-800-HAWORTH, 9:00 a.m. - 5:00 p.m. (EST). E-mail address: docdelivery@haworthpress.com].

The international hospice movement, represented in Botswana, exemplifies a philosophical and service model for multisectoral consideration and implementation on a nationwide scale. The article discusses, inter alia, day care centres and residential units for the terminally ill; a system of highly trained volunteers to work with patients and their families; consistent, skilled nursing services in home based care situations; and halfway houses for training of care-givers as possible solutions to the problem.

The contextualization of such measures will undoubtedly assist in bolstering Botswana's unchallenged record of high standards in governance and social development. *[Article copies available for a fee from The Haworth Document Delivery Service: 1-800-HAWORTH. E-mail address: <docdelivery@ haworthpress.com> Website: <http://www.HaworthPress.com> © 2004 by The Haworth Press, Inc. All rights reserved.]*

KEYWORDS. Home based care, Botswana, HIV/AIDS, ethics, social work-hospice

INTRODUCTION

Home based care (HBC) can be conceptualised and implemented in many different ways; however, as a theoretical concept it should always aim at providing quality care for terminally ill patients and *not* be seen as a solution to overcrowded hospitals. The authors of this article are of the opinion that home based care has the potential to provide patients with the best possible care at home, but that there are limitations which need to be squarely addressed in order to make a national HBC programme a success. Caring for sick people in society and integrating the community in such an activity is not a new concept in Africa, but with the arrival of the AIDS epidemic, the dimensions to care have changed to a degree that government, private sector, and civil society initiatives are urgently needed.

Since the early 1970s, Botswana has based its health policy on the concept of universal health care with an understanding by the Government that access to health care is a basic human right (Government of Botswana & UNDP 1998). The underlying mission has been to provide health care for all, and the country's performance in this regard was exemplary until the HIV epidemic reversed many of the achievements in the health sector. The countries of sub-Saharan Africa generally have the lowest ratio of hospital beds to population in the world, eight to ten times lower than the European average, and scarcer still in rural areas. Special care and longer time frames associated with HIV/AIDS treatment further increase demand for already limited resources (Hope 1999) and, given the scale of the epidemic, Botswana is now a part of this critical situation.

The following argument is based on the assumption that terminally ill patients, in a country like Botswana, should have the right to choose their care environment and that they are entitled to the best possible care available. Currently, patients in Botswana are denied this choice because health workers are obligated to transfer any terminally ill patient to their home if the patient's physical condition allows them to do so, a criterion subject to discursive interpretation. The first part of the paper indicates some of the shortcomings of the current home based care system in Botswana, while the second part discusses alternative and supplementary services that would, it is believed, improve the care given to clients. The authors consider that the current implementation of home based care in Botswana is an unethical solution to the care crisis and argue that appropriate adaptation of the hospice philosophy would improve the situation for all those affected by the epidemic. The role of social workers in this context is examined and suggestions made for their greater involvement in the continuum of care.

THE CONCEPT OF HOME BASED CARE IN BOTSWANA

Conceptually, home based care is a form of community care. In the United Kingdom, for example, community care was officially established as policy in 1990 (the NHS and Community Care Act) to address the needs of the elderly, people suffering from chronic illness, and those living with disabilities (Braye & Preston-Shoot 1996). The key objectives of this model of community care are to promote the development of domiciliary, day care, and respite services to enable people to live in their own homes wherever possible; to ensure that care-givers receive maximum support; and to develop a flourishing independent sector beside quality public programmes through state purchase of services provided by non-governmental organisations (Department of Health 1989).

Domiciliary and day care centre services are available, to a limited extent, in Botswana in the form of home nursing programmes provided by local authorities and non-governmental organisations and a small number of day care centres for the terminally ill. The latter also constitute essential respite services for care-givers. However, a great deal more needs to be done to make home based care a viable alternative to hospital care, especially for HIV/AIDS sufferers and their families. Even in Britain the community care concept has proven to be riddled with complications, exemplified by the observation that

> To the politician community care is a useful piece of rhetoric; to the soci-ologist it is a stick (with which) to beat institutional care . . .; to the civil servant it is a cheap alternative to institutional care which can be passed to the local authorities for action or inaction; to the visionary it is a dream of a new society in which people really do care; to social service departments it is a nightmare of heightened public expectations and in-adequate resources to meet them. (Jones et al., 1978: 114)

However, community home based care is characterised by a number of as-pects that make it a suitable solution in response to the HIV epidemic in a de-veloping country. Since resources are increasingly limited in the public health sector due to the growing number of people falling ill with AIDS related dis-eases, the state is forced to look for alternative ways to care for these clients. In Botswana, according to the 2000 sentinel surveillance, 38.5% of the popula-tion between 15 and 49 years are estimated to be infected with HIV (NACA, AIDS/STD Unit, WHO 2000). Several hospitals currently record that up to 80% of patients in some wards and up to 30% of patients in paediatric wards are hospitalised due to HIV related conditions, while during the period be-tween 1990 and 1996, hospital admissions doubled on a national level (Gov-ernment of Botswana & UNDP 2000). The increasing pressures on the health system have forced health authorities to relocate patients suffering from AIDS related diseases back into the community in order to be able to provide ade-quate care to patients with curable diseases.

The concept of home based care lies at the heart of Botswana's national re-sponse to the epidemic. At the end of June 2000 the cumulative figure for cli-ents registered on home based care stood at 7,000, with the great majority of clients on the programme suffering from AIDS related diseases. Additionally, there is a growing number of children living with an ailing parent or parents and in the year 2000 the number of reported cases was 6,823 (AIDS/STD Unit 2000: 12).

In addition to releasing pressure from hospital facilities, community home based care also has the positive potential to unite aspects of care with preven-tion, which in the past have been commonly treated as two exclusive concepts. By including the family and the community in the care of AIDS patients it be-comes possible to discuss prevention within the community. Once AIDS pa-tients are considered a reality it is easier for people to accept their responsibility to prevent further transmission of the virus (AIDS Action 1995: 2). A view shared by the Government of Botswana:

Caring for patients with AIDS is probably the best way for families and communities to perceive AIDS as a reality in the community and for their own lives. A caring family will also be the best guarantee for prevention of ostracism of people living with HIV/AIDS. (AIDS/STD Unit, Ministry of Health 1996: 4)

Through care in the community, it is thought that the discrimination and isolation of HIV positive people and their families is prevented. However, care within the community should not divert responsibility from the health authority, and there needs to be an understanding that even the institution of the extended family within the African context has its limitations in terms of its ability to care for terminally ill family members (McDonnell et al., 1994: 429).

Also, the ability of the community and the family to provide care needs to be assessed within the economic context of the country and in relation to existing gender imbalances. In regard to the latter, the authors have argued elsewhere that the great majority of carers in Botswana are elderly, and often poor, women while at the same time more women than men are infected with the virus. One could, therefore, argue that the burden of care is placed on the women of Botswana who often live in extremely poor economic conditions (Stegling 2000). Women are generally more affected by poverty than men, making them not only more prone to adopt survival strategies, which might include 'risky' sexual behaviour (Bainame & Letamo 1997: 99) but also making it more difficult for them to look after AIDS patients. Culture also plays a role in the vulnerability of women with regard to risk taking in patient care. This is observed in the unwillingness of many care-givers to wear protective clothing, such as gloves, in the belief that this creates an unacceptable barrier between them and their ailing family members. Social issues surrounding the stigma attached to HIV/AIDS and fear of isolation and alienation by the community also induce high risk behaviours of this nature.

Regardless of the fact that Botswana has recently been classified as a middle income country and that real per capita income increased from US$ 300 in 1966 to US$ 3.300 in 1999, the income poverty rate still stands at about 47% (Government of Botswana & UNDP 2000: 15). In addition, it has been projected that the AIDS epidemic will have a devastating impact on the Gross Domestic Product growth rate mainly due to the loss of skilled labour and increased government expenditure on health and social welfare services.

Home based care should be understood as part of the *continuum of care* a terminally ill patient is receiving. In the case of an AIDS patient, that would be from the time he or she is diagnosed with HIV, and the subsequent counselling, to nutritional advice and emotional support given in order to assist the person while living with the virus but not yet being ill. The care would continue when the person falls ill, ending only when the patient has died. However, a holistic understanding of care for an AIDS patient should also include the emotional support of family members or those who are close to the patient, including the provision of bereavement counselling. Home based care in Botswana needs to be understood as a government organised and formalised programme that has been in place for some time. According to the operational guidelines from the Ministry of Health, support given through government agencies should include counselling of patients and the family at home, material support to assist the carer, continuous visits by health staff, and a monitoring system that co-ordinates the work of the hospital, the clinic, welfare officers, community organisations, and the family. It also acknowledges that carers will need to be trained so that patients receive quality care and carers know how to protect themselves (AIDS/STD Unit 1996).

In some African countries people living with AIDS and their families have benefited from the creation of a continuum of care through the forging of links between patients, their homes, health centres, and district hospitals. In Zambia, Monze District Hospital has developed a community outreach programme including a strong element of support for patients and care-givers in their homes, while the Salvation Army Chikankata Hospital project provides accommodation in the form of traditional houses in the hospital grounds for families of patients so that they can participate in care-giving (Altman 1994). In Uganda, one home based care programme has operationalised the concept of community based support networks comprising lay people, community leaders, and trained community AIDS workers to assist patients and care-givers (Kaya 1999).

Client and Carer Satisfaction with Home Based Care in Botswana

In reality, home based care in Botswana is faced with a number of serious challenges that prevent health care providers from offering the best possible care to those who have fallen ill with AIDS. One of the problems the country is currently facing is that at no time have People Living with HIV and AIDS (PLWHA) been involved in the planning of care services for terminally ill patients (who are, in the context of Botswana, mostly AIDS patients). Even though there are no comprehensive studies available providing data on client satisfaction and care-givers' perceptions on HBC, several smaller research projects have addressed these issues. The following discussion is based on two studies undertaken in March/April 2000 in Kweneng District, Botswana (Khan & Stegling 2000; Mojapelo, Ditirafalo, Tau, & Doehlie 2001).

Both of the studies mentioned earlier identified poverty as the main barrier to the provision of quality care to AIDS patients. In many cases, patients had previously been employed and had contributed significantly to the income of the household. In the first study, of the 29 patients interviewed, 24 had been employed before falling ill, but at the time of the study only 2 were in paid employment. When asked what their main anxieties were, a great majority of patients voiced their concern about the future of their parents or young children after their death, while some were worried about the burden of care which they represented to their families. Many cited, as a major concern, the detrimental effect the disease had on the economic sustainability of the household.

While the government of Botswana provides food and material assistance for clients with terminal illness on home based care, such as a food basket, these services are not always utilised. Since almost all the patients interviewed in this sample denied being HIV positive, they did not utilise certain welfare services because of the stigma attached to these programmes. Their argument was that 'once you receive the food basket, everybody in the community knows that you are an AIDS patient.' Additionally, many patients were unaware of programmes available to them; for example, only a small minority was registered as destitute and the researchers found that, in many cases, only the care-giver was thus nominated, resulting in the entire family sharing one destitute portion which, under the best of circumstances, barely covers the basic needs of one individual (Khan & Stegling 2000: 12-13).

The findings of the second study concurred with those of the first in relation to the patients' experience of poverty; for instance, of the 30 patients interviewed, none was employed at the time of the research. The second study captures very clearly the feelings of patients once they had been discharged on home based care. Even though 39% experienced relief upon discharge, 21% described their emotional state as a feeling of helplessness, a statement that may have been related to the fact that four of the patients did not even have a care-giver when they returned to their homes. Poverty is identified not only by patients as a major problem. It is notably the care-givers who struggle to accommodate patients in a home environment often lacking in basic necessities. Of the care-givers interviewed in the second study, 85% were unemployed and often cited poverty as the main obstacle to the provision of quality care. As one care-giver pointed out:

> *I am suffering because I am poor. I do not have anything to support my patient and myself with. My patient was not working but was able to get a piece job occasionally and we were able to survive.*

Another stated:

> *We need more food and soap. I do not have any clothes myself as well as my patient. We do not have a toilet, we use our neighbour's toilet.*

Furthermore, many care-givers in this study felt unsupported by the extended family and health workers and were, therefore, uncomfortable with the task of looking after an extremely ill patient. Not only did they feel that health care providers were failing to supervise them in their care-taking activity, but also that they, as primary carers, were lacking in medical information to assist them in maintaining high standards of role performance. Below are some of their original statements:

We do not get any assistance from the health workers.

Health workers give us medication only. No other support is provided. Even if the patient is in a bad condition the hospital staff refuse to admit the patient.

My child did not want to be kept in hospital and I was very sad (Kautlwa botlhoko) because of the job involved in caring for the patient at home, cleaning and changing when the patient has diarrhoea. (Mojapelo, Ditirafalo, Tau, & Doehlie 2001)

Another indication of the inadequacy of the home environment is the lack of appropriate shelter. In the second study, two of the patients lived in old derelict houses while one lived in a plastic shack. These are obviously not places where the well-being of patients can be adequately supported. Additionally, as indicated earlier, of the 30 patients interviewed in the second sample, four did not have a care-giver and two were cared for by children, while three had 'care-givers' who were not capable of fulfilling this role due to old age or disability. Furthermore, as stated previously, it should be acknowledged that home based care is not provided by the entire family; in the great majority of cases it is provided by women. Of the 28 care-givers interviewed in the first study all were women, while in the second sample 89% were women. This gender imbalance in the provision of care needs to be addressed, especially since there are currently many voices calling for the greater involvement of men in the fight against AIDS in Botswana.

All these findings indicate that patients are referred home without adequate assessment of their domestic environment despite the fact that, according to the discharge plan utilised in hospitals, social workers should assess the social and economic environment of clients before they are referred (AIDS/STD Unit & WHO 2000). This should not be purported as critical of health workers, since the authors of this article acknowledge that health providers in Botswana are, in many cases, considerably overworked and that most health institutions are faced with a serious problem of under-staffing. In the case of social workers, the current staffing situation is more than dire with some primary hospitals employing one, or at the most, two social workers who are required to conduct all the pre- and post-test counselling in addition to facilitating the referral of patients to home based care. Therefore, the question under debate is whether the system is doing any justice to the increasing number of people falling ill with AIDS. Additionally, there is concern as to whether alternative and supplementary services should be offered to patients in order to maximise the quality of care and to allow for emotional and material support of care-givers and the wider family.

The authors of this paper assert that home based care, as currently implemented in Botswana, possesses unethical implications for patients and care-givers arising out of the system's unrealistic expectations of ordinary people, a great many of whom lack the knowledge, skills, and resources to realise the ultimate goal of home based care, which is to enable death to be experienced in a positive and caring environment of home, family, and friends. Both patient and care-giver (and, indeed, others involved in the situational context) are subjected to symptomatically and circumstantially induced trauma the like of which has not been experienced since the infamous Black Death and other plagues of historical significance, and, on a global scale, never before (Kelly 2001).

THE HOSPICE ALTERNATIVE

One solution to many of the problems associated with home based care in Botswana lies, in the opinion of the writers, in the holistic concept of the international hospice movement whose philosophy, perhaps somewhat ironically, affirms *life* rather than death through providing a place to live rather than to die. It exists to provide support and care for people in the last stages of incurable diseases so that they can live as fully and as comfortably as possible. The hospice concept embraces the belief that, through appropriate care (both physical and psychological) and the development of a concerned community and environment sensitive to the needs of patients and their families, both will be free to attain a degree of mental and spiritual preparation for death (Vancouver Hospice Project unpublished document, cited in Manning 1984).

The theme that unifies all hospice providers around the world is the desire to make available emotional, physical, and spiritual support to patients and their families/care-givers during the course of a terminal illness. In 1975 an international task force established guidelines for hospice programmes based on the following principles:

- Terminally ill people should be accorded control over the dying process.
- Treatment goals should take into account lifestyle and personal preference.
- Family and friends should be assisted in dealing with emotional, financial, and physical stress.
- Physical symptoms of patients should be controlled through programmes of pain relief.
- Hospice staff should be supported in coping with work related stress to help them sustain quality in the performance of their duties (Siebold 1992).

In practical terms, hospice offers services spanning a variety of perspectives and constitutes an ideal environment for an integrated approach to the needs of patients and their families through the co-ordinated efforts of, notably, pastoral, health care, and social work service providers.

Characteristics of Hospice Programmes

Special consideration in such programmes is given to specific factors that characterise the unique nature of hospice. It is the incorporation of these elements that demarcates hospice care from regular hospital services or home based care.

The palliative nature of hospice care focuses on relief from pain and suffering rather than on the curative aspect of treatment. Holistic control of pain and suffering is, in fact, the hallmark of the hospice movement, which espouses the belief that such control should be implicit in all treatment of terminal illness (Manning 1984). The objective is to improve the quality of life through relief measures and better preparation for death.

Demedicalisation of the processes inherent in illness, dying, death, and grief is an integral aspect of hospice service. Categorising conditions (and, by inference, related psycho-social factors) as diseases and pathological states and subsequently treating them as such does little to improve physical, mental, emotional, and psychological health (Siebold 1992). A holistic approach, with emphasis on people taking more responsibility for their own well-being and being supported in this by empathic service providers (including family members), is considered to be a true panacea for pain in all its forms.

In hospice terms, the patient is regarded not as a disease but as a human being experiencing fear, confusion, and anxieties that have to be dealt with in a humane manner by medical and other personnel as well as by care-givers. Open communication is deemed to be vital and, particularly in the residential unit setting, medical staff are always visible, approachable, and willing to discuss any subject that the patient is ready to confront. This is very different from most institutionalised health settings and emphasises the hospice belief that the patient should remain in control of his situation at all times. Death is a stage in the process of personal growth and the dying person is living through the final stage of his/her human condition. During this period life offers the individual a last chance to grow and integrate all dimensions of their existence, to become more human, and to experience a sense of fulfillment (Manning 1984).

In hospice provision, the health care team, comprising the patient, the family, medical, and related staff (including social workers), and volunteers collaborates, through a co-ordinated, multidisciplinary approach, in the provision of quality care. There is a free flow of information and support between all participants and, significantly, even emotional involvement of medical staff with patients, a recognised taboo in traditional medical facilities. In fact, involvement of this nature is the very essence of hospice care (Manning 1984).

Residential hospice units are designed to be as much like home for patients as possible with as few aspects of institutionalisation as is feasible. Because of the nature of terminal illness, hospital-like accommodation might be necessary alongside the care and cluster housing model for those whose condition is not as debilitating. Culture and lifestyle are thus vital considerations in the design of residential services. Home care in ideal circumstances is the zenith of care for the terminally ill but, in many instances, circumstances are not ideal. The strain on families (especially women and especially those in Africa who are considered, unequivocally, to be the primary care-givers) creates an untenable situation for all concerned, including the patient. Even where circumstances in the home allow for quality care, residential hospice provision can be utilised in the short term to ease the sense of responsibility and the pressure on the family during episodes of poor patient health or simply to provide respite to care-givers. Day care programmes also supplement home based care and, where such facilities are attached to residential units, sufferers become familiar with the homely, comforting surroundings, and if admission becomes necessary, proves a less daunting step. There is, in other words, preparation for separation.

Education and training in the management of terminal disease is essential for medical staff who are involved in residential and home based care. Specific courses and in-service lectures, seminars, and workshops on relevant issues instil confidence and allow the staff to investigate their own inner feelings about death and to develop an openness to the feelings of patients regarding *their* mortality. In the process, reticent professionals are transformed into proficient listeners and carers (Kübler-Ross 1969).

An integral component in the process of education and training is supportive supervision of hospice workers and the formation of support groups as vehicles for managing emotional reactions to the demands of the work. Feelings of loss and frustration are commonly addressed in fora such as these. "Working toward good death is rewarding, and it is professionally fulfilling to support one another, especially in sharing burdens and pains brought to the surface, as so often happens, with death and human suffering" (Krant 1974: 97).

Normalising grief is considered essential to enhance the coping mechanisms of families and care-givers. Bereavement and general counselling of family members begins before the death of the patient and is a vital component of hospice service. The human element of the environment, primarily family members and care-givers and *their* needs and feelings, is therefore a highly significant factor in the context of terminal illness and has to be addressed for the sake of the family, as well as that of the patient who might be grappling with a sense of guilt heightened by physical suffering and emotional distress (Manning 1984). Follow-up after the death of the patient is also part of the holistic hospice approach, with support groups for the bereaved playing a significant role in the healing process (Siebold 1992).

Holistic service provision allows for families to be actively and positively involved in (not overwhelmed by) patient care. Even in residential units relatives are encouraged to participate in psychological and physical ministrations to terminally ill family members. Culturally appropriate hospice type villages for families (especially those in which parents and some children may be suffering from HIV/AIDS) as have been established in some African countries, provide income generating projects and employment opportunities for sufferers and their families as well as educational facilities for their children. The concept of family strengthening is an important aspect of hospice service provision in all its forms (Chala 2001).

The welfare of children as patients has a special dimension in the hospice philosophy as childhood, in the natural order, signifies the beginning, rather than the end of life and its potential. Children's residential hospice units in the West provide short term respite or emergency care on behalf of families and care-givers and also permanent services where necessary. In countries such as those on the African continent where AIDS produces large numbers of orphans who may themselves be HIV positive, such units house and care for the children until their death in the belief that a loving, caring, and therapeutic environment prolongs and enhances the quality of life for a sick child.

Hospice in Botswana: Reality and the Road Ahead

Overall, the hospice philosophy incorporates the maxim of death with dignity. This concept arose in the West in the second half of the 20th century largely because of the impersonal, seemingly uncaring institutional approach of large health facilities that prompted the rise of a social movement towards the dignification of the dying process (Siebold 1992). In Africa, death has traditionally been respectfully addressed in customary practice and managed with a high degree of community support and cohesion. The very nature of the AIDS epidemic has, however, denigrated the process and thrust patients and care-givers into dehumanising and degrading situations of physical suffering and stigmatising community response. The "death with dignity" campaign must now be waged on the African front with even greater vigour than in the West, taking into account the scale of the disease and the numbers of people both directly and indirectly affected.

The process has already begun. In Ramotswa (South East District) the Bamelete Lutheran Hospital's hospice programme offers a day care facility for adults, providing opportunities for craftwork, companionship, mutual support, and enhanced nutrition. There is provision for home based care, an in-patient facility in the hospital, nondenominational spiritual care, and bereavement support. Resource persons include nurses, family welfare educators, and trained volunteers. Physical support for home based patient care embraces the provision of adjuncts such as medication, special mattresses, walking aids, and commodes (Kweneng District Multi-Sectoral AIDS Committee 2001).

The Holy Cross Hospice in the capital city, Gaborone, also has an adult day care centre and a home based care service, and organises a volunteer training and service programme. Plans are being formulated for the establishment of a residential unit, which will address the needs of the most serious cases for whom home based care is not a viable option.

The Thirisanyo Catholic Commission provides home based care in Mogoditshane Village on the outskirts of the capital, and is working with Rotary International, UNICEF, the Department of Social Work at the University of Botswana, and SOS Children's Villages to establish a day care centre for pre-school children, an after care centre for school-going children, a recreation centre for out-of-school youth, and a residential facility for homeless children, all of whom are orphans and some of whom will themselves be terminally ill. A drop-in service for HIV positive adults is also being planned. The hospice philosophy is an integral component of this project and will complement its implementation and management. The programme will both employ and network with social workers in much the same manner as the existing SOS Children's Villages in Gaborone and Francistown.

The North East District Multi-Sectoral AIDS Committee, under the auspices of the local authority, has established a day care centre specifically for PLWHA, which caters for approximately thirty people on a daily basis. There is pre-school provision for their children and a drop-in service comprising a counselling/resource centre. The committee has transferred the management of the programme to a community based management trust, which has plans to establish a residential unit in the future. Similar initiatives are being undertaken by other district AIDS committees around the country. As many PLWHA are, in effect, homeless, consideration is also being given to the provision of so-called sheltered accommodation for those who require housing and a certain level of care but are not necessarily in the final stages of terminal illness.[1]

Some districts, such as Kweneng, through their local authorities, are planning the establishment of so-called halfway houses, which will incorporate hospice principles in their service delivery. Notably, patients discharged from hospital to home based care will be accommodated for a period of approximately two weeks, during which time care-givers will be trained in methods of home care. The facility will also provide short term respite services and, in due course, residential care for those in the terminal stages of illness who lack family support, or whose care-givers require assistance (Kweneng District Multi-Sectoral AIDS Committee 2001).

It is the belief of the authors of this article that home based care requires support from government, communities, and non-governmental organisations such as hospice if it is to achieve its objectives. However, it is also our contention that supplementary and alternative services should be given high priority by policy makers and planners in Botswana without delay. Essential to the needs of the country is, in our opinion, the provision of culturally appropriate residential units throughout the country serving as many people as possible, especially those suffering debilitating and dehumanising symptoms (of HIV/AIDS or other terminal or chronic illnesses) and who live under impoverished conditions.

In such contextually relevant residential units or compounds, relatives will be encouraged to spend time with patients and become involved in their physical and psychological care. They will also receive counselling from social workers who will comprise an essential element of the permanent organisational structure, focusing on openness about the illness, the sufferers' feelings, significance of the response of families, and the patients' wishes in regard to their own condition and the future of their children, in particular. In some cases, relatives may be permitted to reside in the unit (especially if travelling distances are great) and arrangements could possibly be made for food to be available for at least one relative per patient. Work with families and outreach and networking services will also constitute an integral element of the social workers' practice. Family villages, as mentioned previously in this article, are another option and could incorporate care-giving of orphaned children by other families participating in the project. Once again, appropriately qualified social workers would be required to co-ordinate and administer welfare services at all levels from a holistic perspective.

Voluntarism, as fostered in the Holy Cross and Bamalete Lutheran Hospice programmes and other home based care services throughout the country, should be encouraged in its purest sense, that is, without material remuneration where possible. Anecdotal evidence suggests that some "volunteers" in Botswana are mainly motivated by the, albeit small, material rewards they receive, which is a denial of the true spirit of voluntarism currently being promoted in the society's war against HIV/AIDS. Some other African countries have a strong tradition of volunteer work, as evidenced by groups such as TASO in Uganda and the Family Health Trust in Zambia (Altman 1994). Student volunteers, popularly utilised in HIV/AIDS programmes in western countries, and others such as Thailand (Lyons 1992), serve the dual purpose of promoting a spirit of community in the youth and addressing the psycho-social needs of terminally ill patients and their families, and should be encouraged in Botswana. The role of social workers in state and non-governmental agencies, within the context of the development of voluntarism within the society, would be to engage in active recruitment and provision of group work services aimed at orientation and training of people of all ages with an interest in community service.

Related to the philosophy of hospice and indirectly aligned to its practice, is the fostering and adoption of children who are known to be HIV positive and thus terminally ill. Botswana is, at present, awaiting the implementation of regulations to the Children's Act of 1981 (which is currently under review) on alternative arrangements for children in need of care, many of whom will be orphans of the AIDS pandemic and possibly infected with the HI virus. This legislation highlights the significance of the social worker's role in the enhancement of adoption and formalised foster care procedures in Botswana with emphasis on *process* and the implicit need for growing numbers of qualified social workers in the provision of alternative care for children. Although the policy stipulates specific testing of children and potential care-givers only in the case of adoption (or permanency planning), where children are known to be HIV positive, adoption and fostering can be arranged in accordance with specific criteria, primarily the provision of in-depth training of alternative care-givers to prepare them for the vicissitudes of placements of this nature (Jacques 1998).

In many industrialised nations the voluntary or non-governmental sector, of which the hospice movement is a part, provides helplines, crisis intervention services, face-to-face counselling, support services for workers involved in HIV/AIDS issues, support groups for families and friends, appropriate housing, and other supplements to home based care. Botswana can and must learn from such models, as indeed is already being demonstrated through the establishment of Lifeline, Childline, and other human rights agencies and programmes. Again, social workers already do, and will continue to, play a major role in the provision of services of this nature.

Policy initiatives for radical responses to the AIDS pandemic must have their roots in lobbying by interest groups at all levels of civil society while government has the responsibility of ensuring their translation into feasible legislative instruments. Social workers, as agents of change in society, play a leading role in this regard both at community and policy making levels. Similarly, financial resources for potential services discussed in this article will emanate from a variety of sources–the state, the private sector, local and international funding agencies, non-governmental organisations, and, possibly, beneficiaries of services themselves through the application of means assessment criteria. The latter procedure is necessitated by the fact that HIV/AIDS, terminal illness generally, dying, death, reluctant or absentee care-givers, and the desire for dignity in the final stages of life are no respecters of income and the ability or inability of clients to purchase services to enhance this period of their lives. However, the concomitant factors of loss of employment, inability to work, and reduction in household income increase the numbers of those requiring financial assistance.

Co-ordination of services and funding mechanisms and procedures are already proving problematic in Botswana's reactive and proactive response to the AIDS pandemic. There is a serious need for strategic planning in this regard with specific emphasis on means of monitoring and evaluation without which essential programmes will flounder and objectives, no matter how pragmatic, will fail to be achieved.

Social work practice, with individuals, families, groups, and communities, and at grassroots and strategic planning levels, will, we hope grow in stature and acceptance and develop a new dimension in a society steeped in the tradition of kinship and a belief in the efficacy of natural support systems. The HIV/AIDS epidemic is fast eroding structures such as these and there is a burgeoning need for professional social work recognition and input to adequately address society's changing demands.

CONCLUSION

The HIV/AIDS pandemic is wreaking havoc in the countries of sub-Saharan Africa, including Botswana, necessitating a variety of traditional and radical responses to stem the tide of the disease and ease the suffering of both infected and affected members of society. The situation in Botswana is, relative to population size, one of the worst in the world and, although awareness is high, specific measures to address needs related to prevention and management are constantly having to be implemented to contain the problem on every front.

Home based care, while politically correct, expedient, and culturally relevant, embodies the germ of exacerbated human suffering for patients and care-givers alike unless rigorously controlled and generously supported through appropriate allocation of material and psycho-social resources. Social workers must be in the forefront of efforts to ensure that this is achieved. Additionally, as the Government of Botswana espouses the provision of universal health care as a basic human right, PLWHA should have the right to choose the care setting they prefer.

The philosophy and practice of the international hospice movement offers meaningful direction in programmes of care for the terminally ill in Botswana and other countries in the region. This is reflected in the Gaborone Declaration, which emanated from the First Regional Southern African Development Community (SADC) Home Based Care Conference held in the Botswana capital in March 2001. The theme of the conference, 'Sharing Responsibilities for Quality Care,' was addressed by delegates from ten SADC countries and the declaration represents consensus on essential principles as foundations for contextualised care of the terminally ill. Concepts include:

- Strengthened community participation and enhancement of the continuum of care.
- Recognition of PLWHA as key stake-holders in programmes of care.
- Improvement of the quality and duration of life.
- Support for care-givers (health care professionals and women).
- Creation of enabling environments through multi-sectoral networks.
- Sustainability of home based care programmes through community involvement.
- Empowerment of patients and families through provision of service options.
- Access to palliative care.
- Development of alternative models of partnerships and programmes.
- Enhancement of support systems.

All these concepts translate into hospice care through which, given political will, effective strategic, fiscal, and operational planning, and a visionary approach, African society may regain agency and once more dare to hope. Social work practitioners are an integral element in the vanguard of success.

NOTE

1. Light and Courage Centre, Francistown. Interview with co-ordinator, June 2001.

REFERENCES

AIDS Action (1995), Issue 28, March-May.

AIDS/STD Unit, Ministry of Health (1996), *Operational Guidelines–Community Home Based Care Programme for People with AIDS in Botswana*/NACP 30, Gaborone.

AIDS/STD Unit, Ministry of Health & World Health Organisation (2000), *A Guide to the Assessment of the Client and Family in Home Based Care*, Gaborone.

AIDS/STD Unit (2000), *Community Home Based Care Newsletter*, Vol. 1, No. 1, Gaborone.

AIDS/STD Unit, Ministry of Health (2001), *Gaborone Declaration on Community Home Based Care*, 1st Regional (SADC) Community Home Based Care Conference, Gaborone.

Altman, D. (1994), *Power and Community: Organisational and Cultural Responses to AIDS*, London: Taylor and Francis.

Bainame, K. & Letamo, G. (1997), *The Socio-Economic and Cultural Context of the Spread of HIV/AIDS in Botswana*, Health Transition Review, Supplement 3, Volume 7, pp. 97-101.

Braye, S. & Preston-Shoot, M. (1996), *Empowering Practice in Social Care*, Buckingham: Open University Press.

Chala, S. (2001), *A Place Where They Can Live and Die with Dignity*, Mail and Guardian, Johannesburg, 9-15 February.

Department of Health (1989), *Caring for People: Community Care in the Next Decade and Beyond*, London: HMSO.

Government of Botswana & United Nations Development Programme (1998), '*Botswana Human Development Report 1997–Challenges for Sustainable Human Development/A Longer Term Perspective,*' Gaborone.

Government of Botswana & United Nations Development Programme (2000), *Botswana Human Development Report 2000: Towards an AIDS-Free Generation*, Gaborone.

Hope, K.R. (1999), The Socio-economic Context of AIDS in Africa: A Review, in Hope, K.R. (Ed.), *AIDS and Development in Africa: A Social Science Perspective*, New York: The Haworth Press, Inc.

Jacques, G. (1998), *Back to the Future: AIDS, Orphans, and Alternative Care in Botswana*. Paper presented at 28th International Conference of Social Welfare, July 5-9, Jerusalem, Israel.

Jones, K., Brown, J. & Bradshaw, J. (1978), *Issues in Social Policy*, London: Routledge and Kegan Paul.

Kaya, H.O. (1999), Beyond the Statistics: HIV/AIDS as a Socio-Economic Epidemic in Africa, Hope, K.R. (Ed.), *AIDS and Development in Africa: A Social Science Perspective*, New York: The Haworth Press, Inc.

Kelly, M.J. (2001), Challenging the Challenger: Understanding and Expanding the Response of Universities in Africa to HIV/AIDS, *Synthesis Report for the Working Group on Higher Education (WGHE)/Association for the Development of Education in Africa (ADEA)*, Washington D. C.: World Bank.

Khan, B. & Stegling, C. (2000), '*Evaluation of the Kweneng District AIDS Home Based Care Programme,*' Unpublished Report for SNV–The Netherlands Development Organisation, Gaborone.

Krant, M.J. (1974), *Dying and Dignity: The Meaning and Control of a Personal Death,* Springfield, Ill.: Charles C Thomas Publishing.

Kübler-Ross, E. (1969), *On Death and Dying,* New York: MacMillan.

Kweneng District Multi-Sectoral AIDS Committee (2001), *Proposal for the Establishment of a Halfway House in Molepolole.*

Lyons, J. (1992), Facing up to AIDS in a Bangkok Slum, Lyons, J. (Ed.), *Community Responses to HIV/AIDS,* New Delhi: UNDP.

Manning, M. (1984), *The Hospice Alternative: Living with Dying,* London: Souvenir Press.

McDonnell, S., Brennan, M., Burnham, G. & Tarantola, D. (1994), *Assessing and Planning Home Based Care for Persons with AIDS,* Health Policy and Planning, Vol. 9, No. 4, pp. 429-437.

Mojapelo, D., Ditirafalo, T., Tau, M. & Doehlie, E. (2001), *Client Satisfaction and Providers' Perspectives of Home Based Care in Kweneng District,* Botswana, Unpublished Report, Gaborone.

National AIDS Co-ordinating Agency, AIDS/STD Unit, World Health Organisation (2000), *Botswana 2000 HIV Sero-prevalence and STD Syndrome Sentinel Survey, Technical Report,* Gaborone.

Siebold, C. (1992), *The Hospice Movement: Easing Death's Pains,* New York: Twayne Publishers.

Stegling, C. (2000), *Current Challenges of HIV/AIDS in Botswana,* Working Paper, No. 1, Department of Sociology, University of Botswana, Gaborone.

Stegling, C. (2000), *AIDS Home Based Care and Female Poverty in Botswana,* Mmegi/The Reporter, 01-07 September, Gaborone.

FROM DUAL DIVISIONS TO HUMAN RIGHTS: CONSTRUCTING A HOLISTIC APPROACH TO MENTAL HEALTH

Mental Health Practice and Children: Dogma, Discourse, Debate, and Practice

Barbara Fawcett

SUMMARY. In the field of mental health, debates range along opposing axes with the protection of the public on one axis and the citizenship and human rights of the individual on the other. There is also considerable contestation for ideological and theoretical dominance about how mental distress should be viewed and responded to. Discourses alternatively emphasising protection, control and compulsion, and rights, citizenship autonomy and self-determination have added impetus when applied to

Barbara Fawcett, PhD, is Head of Department of Social Sciences and Humanities, University of Bradford, West Yorkshire, BD7 1DP, UK (E-Mail: B.H.Fawcett1@bradford.ac.uk).

[Haworth co-indexing entry note]: "Mental Health Practice and Children: Dogma, Discourse, Debate, and Practice." Fawcett, Barbara. Co-published simultaneously in *Social Work in Mental Health* (The Haworth Social Work Practice Press, an imprint of The Haworth Press, Inc.) Vol. 2, No. 2/3, 2004, pp. 195-206; and: *Social Work Approaches in Health and Mental Health from Around the Globe* (ed: Metteri et al.) The Haworth Social Work Practice Press, an imprint of The Haworth Press, Inc., 2004, pp. 195-206. Single or multiple copies of this article are available for a fee from The Haworth Document Delivery Service [1-800-HAWORTH, 9:00 a.m. - 5:00 p.m. (EST). E-mail address: docdelivery@haworthpress.com].

Digital Object Identifier: 10.1300/J200v2n02_12

children and young people. This is also a grouping denied a voice both in terms of individual treatment programmes and in the formulation of policy and practice. This article addresses the key debates and appraises the implications of changing policy and practice for children and young people experiencing mental distress in the UK. Although the discussion is located in a particular national context, the emergent themes have a much broader relevance for debates, policy and practice in the international arena. *[Article copies available for a fee from The Haworth Document Delivery Service: 1-800-HAWORTH. E-mail address: <docdelivery@haworthpress.com> Website: <http://www.HaworthPress.com> © 2004 by The Haworth Press, Inc. All rights reserved.]*

KEYWORDS. Mental health, children, young people, medicalisation, user involvement

INTRODUCTION

In the United Kingdom, mental health services for children and young people are described as under resourced, inadequately staffed, fragmented and ill equipped to deal with the needs of children and young people (Young Minds 2000; Mental Health Foundation, 2001). More government money is being allocated, but problems remain. This article begins by providing a backdrop to the current situation concerning children and young people in the United Kingdom by looking at debates and policy initiatives in the field of adult mental health services. It then interrogates current provision for children and young people by highlighting problem areas before moving on to discuss possible ways forward.

THE CONTEXT: ADULT MENTAL HEALTH SERVICES

The arena of 'mental health' has long been beset by competing discourses, each highlighting different ways of conceptualising and responding to the situation as differentially defined. Models highlighting aspects relating to health and defining problems as illnesses with symptoms that can be categorised and treated predominantly, but not exclusively, with drug and physical treatments (for example, Linford Rees, 1978; Howe, 1995) have been set against more socially oriented models, which focus on removing stigma, stressing citizenship rights and promoting a broader based response to mental distress/'madness' (e.g., Rogers and Pilgrim, 1996, 1999; Prior, 1993; Sayce, 2000; Beresford, 2000). The very terminology used highlights differential discursive allegiances. The use of terms relating to mental ill health or illness, for example, firmly locate discussions within medicalised frames of reference. Terms such as 'mental distress' broaden the conceptual range, placing difficulties experienced on a continuum where it is acknowledged that we all experience problems at various points in time with some being more severe than others. There is also the use of the originally pejorative term 'madness' reused and revalued as a positive statement of difference to consider. Commentators such as Rachel Perkins (1999) present the view that minimising difference via the apparently inclusive language of distress is unhelpful and illusory. Passing as 'sane' and denying difference is seen to perpetuate oppression. Perkins (1999) insists (and in this she draws from black and lesbian/gay politics) that real inclusion can be achieved only by the celebration of difference and diversity and maintains: 'so let's dispense with notions of distress and embrace mad pride' (Perkins, 1999, p. 6). However, despite varying interpretations and differing terminology, it would be unhelpful to suggest that the discursive interpretations (although sometimes presented as such) are mutually exclusive. There is considerable overlap, although it is important to highlight that medicalised perspectives in relation to both adult services and those for children and young people retain dominance in relation to resources, services and policy.

In the United Kingdom, policy is changing rapidly in the field of 'mental health.' The White Paper 'Modernising Mental Health Services' (1998), the National Service Framework for Mental Health (2000) and the proposed reform of the 1983 Mental Health Act, which specifies how people diagnosed as suffering from a 'mental disorder' can be compulsorily detained, have all made a significant contribution.

'Modernising Mental Health Services' (1998) focuses on the improved assessment of individual needs, better treatment and care both at home and in hospital and access to services on a twenty-four hour basis. There is a predominant emphasis on ensuring public safety and managing risk and upon mental health services being based in primary care with close links being maintained with specialist teams to integrate service planning and delivery. Close partnerships are envisaged with education, employment and housing departments. The need for patients, service users and carers being involved in their own care and in planning services is also highlighted. Services are to be delivered in the most efficient cost effective way with clear guidance from the National Institute for Clinical Excellence. There is also a commitment to improve secure hospital services with public protection remaining a first priority at all times.

The National Service Framework for Mental Health (2000) focuses on strengthening partnerships across National Health Service and social care organisations. The Framework incorporates standards relating to five main areas. These are mental health promotion; primary care and access to services; services for people with severe mental illness; support for carers; and the prevention of suicide. The standards are linked to existing statistics, and milestones and performance indicators have been specified in order to measure progress.

The proposed reform of the Mental Health Act 1983 looks to modernise services by facilitating compulsory treatment taking place in the community as part of an agreed care plan. This is highly controversial and again demonstrates a focus on drug therapies and the importance of prioritising the protection of the public over service user choice. The new provisions also remove the independent non-clinical role of the Approved Social Worker. Under the current legislation in the United Kingdom, the Approved Social Worker decides whether an application for compulsory detention in hospital ought to be made and whether detention in hospital is, taking into account all the circumstances, the most appropriate way of providing the care and treatment that the person needs. The new proposals allow the application to be made by a suitably trained mental health professional, thus and again controversially, reverting to the sole involvement of clinicians in relation to compulsory treatment (Reforming the Mental Health Act 2001; Karban, 2001).

Current policy highlights the need for intensive and extensive support for people experiencing mental health difficulties. It focuses on the need to reduce stigma and emphasises the importance of including service users and carers in planning processes. More resources to mental health services are also to be made available subject to cost effectiveness and gate keeping mechanisms. However, the policy documents clearly view problems with mental health in terms of requiring medical treatment and stress the importance of controlling those assessed as possibly unpredictable or violent and the need to care for those regarded as vulnerable. 'Control' and 'care' are terms that have featured significantly in the welfare literature and these are terms vociferously rejected by proponents of more socially oriented models of mental distress (Sayce, 2000). Indeed, there can be seen to be clear tensions in policy frameworks which advocate care and control on the one hand and partnership, service user involvement and social inclusion the other.

Additional tensions in relation to current policy initiatives are also evident. With regard to the provision of citizenship rights, in the United Kingdom (and indeed elsewhere) responsibilities are being emphasised as a pre-requisite for the exercise of rights. This makes it difficult for those diagnosed (in accordance with dominant medical model frameworks) to achieve enduring rights of citizenship. A further tension can be associated with the setting of a national service framework for mental health and the identification and promotion of national standards and competencies. Undoubtedly, the setting of standards nationally to be delivered locally and monitored externally with the National Service Framework setting out service blueprints, sounds both proactive and positive. Targetting services and relating specific professional competencies to services can ensure that previously marginalized areas are better resourced and that good practice standards are maintained. However, it can also serve to exclude those who do not fit service criteria and to discourage locally relevant and innovative forms of provision. It can also re-inforce the view that professionals have to prioritise covering themselves at the expense of meeting the individual needs of service users and carers. The agenda of controlling outcomes does not fit with service user self-determination.

The policy documents also insufficiently differentiate between the self-assessed needs of service users and those of carers. As with previous policies in the field, there is an emphasis on carers views taking precedence over the expressed wishes of individuals diagnosed as mentally ill. Modernising Mental Health Services (4.50) states:

> Decisions about care and treatment should be a joint endeavour between staff, patients, service users and discussed with carers as well. Carers are partners alongside health and social services in providing care and support to people with mental health problems.

This links into debates about the modernising agenda and its underlying rationality. The Government promotes policies as being modern and rational. There is an emphasis on order and on the rational, linear progression of policy into practice. Service users are located within a clear diagnosis-treatment continuum and subject to expert-patient relationships. Rhetoric about patients being 'informed, involved, and empowered' seems to translate into being consulted rather than having any real control or being able to exercise autonomy about the making of decisions that affect their lives.

POLICIES AND PRACTICES FOR CHILDREN AND YOUNG PEOPLE

A key question to ask at this point is where children and young people fit in relation to current debates and the prevailing policy and practice framework. It is interesting to note that both 'Modernising Mental Health Services' (1998) and the Government's National Service Framework for Mental Health (2000) specifically excludes services for children and adolescents. Services for this group come under the heading of Child and Adolescent Mental Health Services (CAMHS). The government in the United Kingdom is committed to increase the amount of funding made available, but to date money made available has not been ringfenced. There are also plans to bring CAMHS into the National Service Framework for Children in 2003.

As highlighted in the introduction, Child and Adolescent Mental health Services have been described as 'fragmented, patchy, and unsatisfactory' (Young Minds, 2000 p. 7). Recommendations made include the need for more specialists in patient provision, the strengthening of specialist community based services, the inclusion of children and young people with mental health problems within the National Service Framework for Mental Health and the improved co-ordination of services. Now on one level, these recommendations are perfectly acceptable. However, on another they raise a number of issues that relate to children and young people seen to have mental health problems. These issues will now be discussed as it can be argued that these have a wider ranging relevance.

A key issue relates to the fact that discussions focusing on the mental health of children and young people are firmly located within medicalised discourses. As discussed earlier, medicalised discourses view problems with mental health as illnesses that require specialist diagnosis and treatment. There are positive factors related to medicalised perspectives. These can provide frameworks that enable a 'person in chaos' who perceives themselves or who is perceived by others to be experiencing difficulties (Bracken & Thomas, 2000) to order what is going on for them. Medicalised frameworks can also enable a person (and their family) not to feel that what is happening is their fault. An individual is not seen as responsible for their actions and there are services and professionals to call upon to intervene to provide relief for families and drug and therapeutic forms of relief for an individual. Policies, services, and resources can also be directed towards an identified, particularly vulnerable group, who require both care and control.

However, there are also negative factors. Medicalised frameworks, for example, can provide explanations and treatment framework that negate other possibilities. Such approaches can result in a failure to explore reasons for pain, suffering and disturbed behaviour and the context in which it is manifested. A focus on pathology can also simplify and reduce an individual's experiences and an emphasis on expert intervention can control and disempower individuals.

Bracken and Thomas (2000) assert

> most psychiatric diagnoses are nothing more than a particular way of formulating and naming a person's problems. . . . Psychiatric diagnosis is often little more than a simplification of a complex reality, and by for-

mulating an individual's experiences in terms of pathology it can be profoundly disempowering and stigmatising. (p. 19)

User or survivor movements, aligned to shifts in social theorising, have rejected the notion that there is an objective, value free continuum that moves clearly through a symptom–diagnosis–treatment–cure–continuum. The work of Fernando (1993), Pilgrim and Rogers (1997), Sayce (2000), Bracken and Thomas (2000) to name but a few, have highlighted that unacknowledged cultural, social, economic, and ideological assumptions and value systems render any claims to objectivity obsolete. From an historical perspective, a review of nineteenth century concepts of psychiatry, particularly in relation to how these refer to women, highlight how relative 'facts' can be. An example, mentioned in Showalter (1985) shows how Henry Maudsley, an eminent Victorian psychiatrist and professor, both reflected and promoted the view, portrayed as fact, that mental activity in women affected their menstrual cycle resulting in serious illnesses such as epilepsy or marital breakdown. Beresford (2001) calls for 'non-medicalised alternatives' for children and criticises 'an outmoded psychiatric system that still frequently fails to see the person and only sees the illness.' He goes on to say that 'in doing so, it misses both people's strengths and their difficulties' (Beresford 2001, p. 14).

Another area to highlight is that children and young people can be experiencing similar difficulties, but be responded to in a variety of different ways. With regard to problem identification and associated responses, initially an area has to be identified as a problem by a child, young person, family, professional or school, and action has to be deemed to be necessary. Different children, young people and families will view similar problems very differently. Some will find themselves in crisis and require emergency intervention, some will seek assistance and some will manage the problem or difficulty themselves. Additionally, the same problem can be directed to a variety of agencies and professionals and be responded to in a variety of different ways. The same problem could, for example, be directed towards a social services department, a voluntary agency, the police, the courts, the education services, general practitioners, psychologists, or psychiatrists. In each instance a different response could be obtained. There is also wide variation in terms of when a difficulty or problem becomes a condition: For example, when high activity in a child becomes a hyperkinetic disorder, when challenging behaviour becomes a conduct disorder, and when a child having an imaginary friend becomes 'hearing voices,' which is then translated into early onset schizophrenia.

There is additionally wide divergence about which difficulties constitute a mental health emergency. Some agencies refuse to consider a referral if drugs or alcohol are involved (Street, 2000). Some regard 'challenging behaviour' as being within the remit of CAMHS, others regard it as being outside. There are wide differences in the age of transition between children's and adult services with some effecting the transition at 16 and some at 19. There are also differences in the identification and prevalence of mental health disorders according to the social class of the father. According to Kurtz (1996) children and young people from social class five (unskilled) are three times more likely to be diagnosed with mental health problems than those in social class one. This leads to the classic question about whether greater stressors (e.g., life in an inner city) result in greater mental health problems or whether professionals are more likely to diagnose difficulties as mental health problems for those living in inner cities.

A third issue relates to a lack of focus on what children and young people want and would find helpful. Very few services and studies have actually asked children and young people what they want. Two notable exceptions, which have concentrated upon children and young people in the 16- to 25-year age group, are The Mental Health Foundation (1999), and The Mental Health Foundation (2001). The Mental Health Foundation Report published in 2001 entitled 'Turned Upside Down' (Smith and Leon, 2001) highlights that young people feel intimidated by psychiatrists and largely find general practitioners unhelpful. In the study that informed the report, the views of forty-five young people with experience of mental health crises were explored using questionnaires, face-to-face interviews and focus groups. The young people involved in the study talked about not being listened to; about not being heard and supported; and having to meet tightly defined criteria that excluded many of them when seeking help (MHF 2001, p. 30). Young people emphasised the importance of services being able to

- Listen to and understand young people
- Allow and encourage young people to talk and explain their situation
- Provide help and advice
- Be respectful of their situation
- Employ a range of staff with experience of mental health problems
- Facilitate and provide support groups
- Offer confidentiality
- Involve young people

As highlighted, research currently portrays Child and Adolescent Mental Health Services as being in crisis (Young Minds, 2000; Mental Health Foundation, 2001). However, a key question to pose relates to how should services be developed. Should there be a continuation of existing services, but with improved resources; should there continue to be a predominant medical orientation; should there be a shift to a social orientation; or should emphasis be placed on a flexible, accessible, young person centred combination. Given the comments made by young people themselves, perhaps it is the latter that currently carries most weight. It is also not a question of posing a simplistic dichotomy between social and medical orientations, but of deconstructing and reconstructing terms such as 'children and young person centred,' 'involvement,' 'participation,' and 'multidisciplinary.' As part of the deconstruction process, the ways in which these terms are currently used in varying contexts would have to be explored and the implications for the different participants or stakeholders examined. Part of the reconstruction could include the formulation of clear principles upon which services could be based. Such principles would have to be frequently reviewed by children, young people and the other participants involved in service planning and service delivery, to prevent fixed, rigid interpretations, which over time could subvert their very purpose.

A key principle would have to evolve around an emphasis on trust and confidentiality, with the child or young person being fully involved in any process with this including being able to give or withhold consent. This is controversial, but participation without such safeguards is unlikely to fully engage and maintain the position of the child or young person at the centre of the activity. This then raises issues which can best be referred to as 'what if' scenarios. What if the child or young person is out of control, what if they are likely to harm themselves, what if they are likely to harm others, what if they have already harmed themselves and/or others. Perhaps, a key response to such scenarios is to highlight a second key principle, which is about placing emphasis on working with the child/young person's definition of the situation. Research shows that professionals consistently highlight difficulties in working with those who refuse to engage (Kurtz et al., 1995; Howarth and Street, 2000; Young Minds, 2000). It can be argued that unless those operating in the field of child and adolescent mental health appropriately engage with the child/young person in a way that they understand, focus on what they think is happening and what (if anything) they want to do about it, then little is going to be achieved. Research reviewed by Featherstone and Parton (2001) in relation to child protection leads the authors to state 'The child protection system as it currently operates does not appear to be invested in by those whom it is set up to protect' (Featherstone and Parton, Working Paper, p. 25). They point to the very different understandings of the term 'safe' held by adults (parents and professionals) and children and young people. For adults, 'safe' means parents/professionals acting in what they believe to be the child or young person's best interests. However, young people see 'safe' to mean confidentiality and maintaining control over what happens to them. This means confiding in peers, not adults, if there is a fear of losing control over events. In this context, the work of Featherstone and Parton (2000) has a strong relevance for child and adolescent mental health services. It also highlights that there can be clear divergences between the agendas of children and young people, parents, and professionals. This leads into a discussion about rights. The United Nations Convention on Rights of the Child Article 12 dealing with the 'Right of Participation' draws attention to children and young people having the right to express their views in all matters affecting them. With regard to current policies, the 1989 Children Act in the UK also emphasises the importance of listening to children. The Social Exclusion Unit's Policy Action Team's Report on Young People (2000) also stresses the need to design policies around the needs and priorities of young people. Similarly, the Connexions initiative related to the 13-19-year-old age group recommends that each young person involved in the initiative requires a personal advisor to help with information, advice and support and to facilitate access to specialist services if required. There is also the enactment of the Human Rights Act 1998 in the United Kingdom to consider. Human Rights legislation can criticise local authorities for failing to act to protect children as occurred in the Bedfordshire case (European Court of Human Rights, Strasbourg 2001) or can emphasise rights to involvement and participation depending upon the interpretation given to the different Articles. However, the point to be made here is that children and young people do have rights (arguably they should have more), and that these have to be looked at very carefully and prioritised in relation to resource allocation and service development.

In line with the principles highlighted here a range of services could be developed and existing services further developed relating to what children and young people say they want and would find useful. These would include a wide range of community oriented, fully resourced, user friendly services. Spandler (1996) and the Mental Health Foundation (2001) report children and young people wanting directly accessible non-clinical, confidential, flexible, non-compulsory services available on a twenty-four hour basis. Interestingly, there is also an emphasis on such services being staffed by those who have experienced similar problems themselves. E-mail and Internet services also feature, as do self-access confidential counselling services and independent advocacy services. Full information and publicity for all services is also recommended. When a child or young person is experiencing very severe or constantly reoccurring crises, supported access to user friendly, intensive support services are emphasised. All services would need ongoing 'action evaluations' by all those involved (see Fawcett, 2000) with findings continually feeding into service development.

It can be argued that there should be clear differentiation between the involvement of children and young people and that services should develop differently to meet the needs of these two diverse groupings. The situation with regard to younger children is contentious and the case for the involvement of an independent advocate can be clearly made. However, it can be argued that in terms of the development of key principles and accessible supportive, flexible services, similar points can be made for both children and young people.

CONCLUSION

Movement is taking place in relation to service user involvement and the exercise of autonomy and control with regard to adult services. As Roberts (2000) asserts, the disability movement and its emphasis on overcoming social, economic, and political barriers to the achievement of full inclusive citizenship rights and eschewing pathologising and objectifying classifications has influenced survivor movements two decades younger. However, it is important to point out that although disabled people have been involved in writing the Disability Discrimination Act 1995 in the UK and the United Nations Standard Rules and the Declaration of Rights of Disabled Persons, 'survivors' of the mental health system have not been involved in reform of the Mental Health Act (1983) in the UK (Roberts, 2000; Bracken and Thomas, 2000). Prioritisation also continues to be given in a routinised manner to the protection of the public over the rights of the individual experiencing mental health difficulties.

In this article, it has been argued that issues relating to autonomy and control need to be addressed with regard to Child and Adolescent Mental Health Services. In the UK, CAMHS can be seen to have reached a crossroad and there is the opportunity to radically overhaul and develop initiatives and projects that are responsive to the stated needs of those concerned. This is not to set service users against practitioners. Both can constructively work together to produce policies and services that children and young people can positively and productively invest in.

REFERENCES

Audit Commission (1999) Children in Mind, London.

Barnes, R. and Bowl, M. (2001) Taking over the Asylum–Empowerment and Mental Health, Basingstoke, Palgrave.

Beresford, P. (2001) 'Removing the Pain' in Community Care 7-13th June 2001, p. 14.

Bracken, P. and Thomas, P. (2001) 'Evidence-Based Medicine and Advocacy' in Openmind 107 Jan/Feb 2001, p. 19.

Department of Health People Like Us: The Report of the review of the Safeguards for children Living Away From Home, Sir William Utting, London, HMSO.

Department of Health (1998) Modernising Mental Health Services, London, HMSO.

Department of Health (1999) National Service Framework: Mental Health, London, HMSO.

Fawcett, B. (2000) Feminist Perspectives on Disability, Harlow Prentice Hall.

Featherstone, B. and Parton N. (2001) Placing Children Centrally in Child Protection, Working paper, University of Huddersfield.

Fernando, S. (1993) Mental Health, Race and Culture, Basingstoke, Macmillan/Mind.

Howarth, C. and Street, C. (2000) Sidelined: Young Adults' Access to Services, London, New Policy Institute.

Howe, G. (1995) Working with Schizophrenia: A Needs Based Approach, London, Jessica Kingsley.

Karban, K. (2001) Social Work and Mental Health: The End or a New Beginning, article in progress.

Kurtz, Z., Thornes, R. and Wolkind, S. (1995) Services for the Mental Health of Children and Young People in England: Assessment of Needs and Unmet Need, London, Public Health Directorate, South Thames RHA.

Kurtz, Z. (1996) Treating Children Well, London, The Mental Health Foundation.

Linford Rees, W.L. (1978) A Short Textbook of Psychiatry, Second Edition, London, Hodder and Stoughton.

Perkins, R. (1999) 'Madness, distress, and the language of inclusion' in OpenMind 98, July/August 1999.

Pilgrim D. and Rogers, A. (1999) A Sociology of Mental Health and Illness, Second Edition, Buckingham, Open University Press.

Prior, L. (1993) The Social Organisation of Mental Illness, London, Sage.

Roberts, M. (2000) 'Come Together? Right Now?' in Openmind, No. 106 Nov/Dec 2000, p. 12.

Sayce, L. (2000) From Psychiatric Patient to Citizen: Overcoming Discrimination and Social Exclusion, Basingstoke, Macmillan.

The Mental Health Foundation (1999) Bright Futures, London, The Mental Health Foundation.

The Mental Health Foundation (2001) Turned Upside Down: Developing Community-Based Crisis Services for 16-25 Year Olds Experiencing a Mental Health Crisis, Smith, K. and Leon, L., London, The Mental Health Foundation.

Young Minds (2000) Whose Crisis: Meeting the Needs of Children and Young People with Serious Mental Health Problems, Street, C., London, Young Minds.

Youth Access (2001) Breaking Down the Barriers: Key Evaluation Findings on Young People's Mental Health Needs, London, Youth Access/Department of Health.

Social Exclusion and Psychosis:
Exploring Some of the Links
and Possible Implications for Practice

Helen Barnes

SUMMARY. This article considers aspects of the possible impact of social exclusion upon psychosis and the implications of this for mental health social work practice. Against a background of calls for evidence based practice, and increasing recognition of the significance of theories and understandings as the foundations of practice, the article will first explore current and historical ways of viewing and intervening with the relationship between social adversity and mental health. Then, alternative understandings of this relationship, supported by recent research regarding the impact of trauma and extreme social adversity upon physiological and physical processes implicated in mental ill-health, will be discussed. These approaches have major implications for social work practice with psychosis, suggesting that experiences of trauma and disadvantage, and interventions seeking to alleviate the inner and outer effects of these experiences–tasks central to the social work remit–can make a significant difference to mental health outcomes. However, this

Helen Barnes, BA(Hons), PhD, CQSW, is Senior Lecturer in Social Work, Staffordshire University, Institute of Social Work and Applied Studies, Brindley Building, Leek Road, Stoke on Trent, Staffordshire, ST4 2DF, UK (E-mail: barnes.h@staffs.ac.uk).

[Haworth co-indexing entry note]: "Social Exclusion and Psychosis: Exploring Some of the Links and Possible Implications for Practice." Barnes, Helen. Co-published simultaneously in *Social Work in Mental Health* (The Haworth Social Work Practice Press, an imprint of The Haworth Press, Inc.) Vol. 2, No. 2/3, 2004, pp. 207-233; and: *Social Work Approaches in Health and Mental Health from Around the Globe* (ed: Metteri et al.) The Haworth Social Work Practice Press, an imprint of The Haworth Press, Inc., 2004, pp. 207-233. Single or multiple copies of this article are available for a fee from The Haworth Document Delivery Service [1-800-HAWORTH, 9:00 a.m. - 5:00 p.m. (EST). E-mail address: docdelivery@haworthpress.com].

Digital Object Identifier: 10.1300/J200v2n02_13

is not to advocate a simple (albeit under-resourced) 'social solution'! On the contrary, the understandings underpinning these approaches recognise biological processes play a role in mental and physical ill-health: importantly, however, they can be shown to question the stigma traditionally attached to the concept of biological disorder in mental health, thus pointing to the value of a truly biopsychosocial approach with psychosis, involving fully holistic interventions that differ from those currently dominant, and which carry implications for more egalitarian worker-user relationships. *[Article copies available for a fee from The Haworth Document Delivery Service: 1-800-HAWORTH. E-mail address: <docdelivery@haworthpress.com> Website: <http://www.HaworthPress.com> © 2004 by The Haworth Press, Inc. All rights reserved.]*

KEYWORDS. Mental health, psychosis, social exclusion, social work, sociological realism, enduring serious mental health problems, psychobiology, trauma, poverty, biopsychosocial approach

INTRODUCTION

There has been increasing attention in national (e.g., Great Britain: Department of Health 1999b; 2001) and international (World Health Organisation 2001) policy to links between the social environment, social exclusion, and health, with strong evidence that much higher rates of both mental and physical ill-health are found amongst socially excluded groups (Acheson 1998, Duggan 2002, Henderson et al., 1998). Statham (2000) has highlighted the importance of the widespread policy emphasis on partnership between health and social care agencies in addressing these links, and there are new calls for evidence based practice in social work and social care (Great Britain: Department of Health 2000). This focus of attention promises to provide significant opportunities for social work to develop a more prominent role in mental health work, but what shape can this role take?

Howe (1987) has shown that interventions with health and welfare problems (or indeed with any problems) are based on theories and understandings about how the problems have arisen, and those interventions will be more effective to the extent that those understandings are grounded in research into the nature of the problems. This is a very topical issue with regard to the links between physical and mental ill-health and the social environment, for the nature of these links has not been well-understood (World Health Organisation 2001, Duggan 2002), and social work has often had a limited engagement with them (Bywaters & McLeod 1996).

Beliefs influencing policy and practice may often come not only from formal or professional theories, but from societal theories, operating at a tacit level in people's consciousness (Thompson 2000a)–theories we need to make explicit and question if we are to practice effectively and responsively. This articles therefore, seeks to explore some of the understandings, societal and professional, that currently appear to underpin practice with people with enduring serious mental health problems and their experiences of social exclusion, and to look at what recent research can tell us about the way these experiences can impact on mental health–and in particular psychosis. By exploring some of these links, we can consider possibilities for the role of mental health social work in health and social care partnerships working with serious mental health problems.

LEGACY OF HISTORY FOR MENTAL HEALTH PRACTICE

Social Exclusion Yesterday and Today

Social exclusion has been identified as exclusion from citizenship–'the civil and political rights and obligations, that all members of society should have' (Giddens 1998, pp. 102-3). From the 'Enlightenment' period in Western industrialised societies to today, in these societies, exclusion from such rights and obligations–e.g., participation, employment, social engagement–has been connected inextricably to poverty and stigma (Golding and Middleton 1982, Gordon et al., 2000, Becker 1997), and people with enduring serious mental health problems have been particularly likely to be in this position then and now (Scull 1983, Thornicroft 1993, Dunn 1999). Significantly, Bracken and Thomas (2001) have suggested that current policy and practice in respect of the latter group is informed by beliefs emanating from the Enlightenment period. What, then, may be the legacy of these historical understandings about social exclusion and psychosis for practice today?

Citizenship and the Enlightenment

The Enlightenment in eighteenth century Europe bequeathed to us with massive implications for much of the world, the belief, articulated by the philosophers Kant and Descartes, that the essence of the human being lay in the faculty of 'reason'–the ability to perceive and understand a situation, think about it, and problem-solve. Later, in the nineteenth century, Darwin developed his highly influential theory of evolution, portraying humans with well-developed 'reason' as at the top of the evolutionary hierarchy, having the capacity to adjust and survive (O'Brien and Penna 1998).

Within this belief system, a great division was perceived between humans, ruled by 'mind' and 'reason,' and animals ruled by their biology, and desires, impulses or emotions. Animals and the environment were classed as 'nature,' beings that simply existed, while 'man' with his reasoning and problem solving capacities was thought in contrast to be as God–capable of controlling the material, natural and social worlds (O'Brien and Penna 1998). In the human, therefore, Darwin saw the emotions as an 'archaic remnant' (Williams 1998).

Through 'reason' therefore, the individual was expected to be independent, autonomous: In the newly industrialised societies of the 'Enlightenment,' the efficient working of society was thought to be dependent on this. Industry organised to make profits for its owners required individuals to be highly skilled and self-disciplined at work, and without the controls of close traditional communities they had to be able to control their own behaviour if social order was to be maintained (Cuff 2000). This meant being in control of 'nature' outside them in work (the material environment) and inside them in the community (their emotions, bodies, and impulses)–Ingleby (1983). The individual who achieved this was seen as 'proprietor of his own person and capacities, owing nothing to society for them' (MacPherson 1962, p. 3, cited in Dalley 1988, p. 28) and in these societies, it was only such highly functioning individuals who could access social inclusion: Only they could obtain employment, and through this a wage–which in these societies organised to deter people from voluntary unemployment (O'Brien and Penna 1998), formed the only means of purchasing life's needs–and citizenship rights.

Mental Health

Against this background, mental health, defined as the healthy mind with the capacities of 'reason' necessary for the person to 'strive' for active logical and ethical adaptation to the environment' (World Health Organisation 1955, p. 12), has been seen as essential for the good working of society. The mentally healthy person has thus been understood to possess:

- Balance of psychic forces (emotions not dominating)
- Resistance to stress
- Autonomy
- Competence
- Perception of reality

(Jahoda 1958)

Mental ill-health has therefore been seen as a failure in these capacities of 'mind' and 'reason,' cast in Enlightenment thought as the product of abnormality in the inner workings of the individual (Bracken & Thomas 2001). These problems of poor mental functioning are expected to result in difficulties in performing social roles. There is, then, no place in industrial societies, where so much importance is placed on the individual's competence and self-control, for these people, perceived widely in society as 'backward' and 'amoral' (Furnham & Rees 1988) out of control of both their outer and their inner worlds.

In earlier times, this meant people with serious mental health problems were amongst the poor and homeless (Scull 1983; Ripa 1990); they then were excluded through incarceration in the asylums found in many western countries in the 1800s onwards (Rogers & Pilgrim 2001), and then with deinstitutionalisation returned to societies and employment systems still organised around individuals with maximum functioning (Oliver 1996) thus encountering social exclusion in the community once again. As a result, community care services have acknowledged both health and social care needs, thus recognising and responding, to some extent, to barriers denying these groups rights and an acceptable life in the community (Hyde 2000), but ultimately, these barriers are thought to be the product of their own poor functioning.

How, then, is the relationship between mental health and social exclusion understood in current policy and practice? We will consider this, and then explore alternative perspectives drawing on recent research evidence, which appear to carry substantial and meaningful implications for social work with people experiencing psychosis.

CURRENT UNDERSTANDINGS OF MENTAL HEALTH AND SOCIAL EXCLUSION IN POLICY AND PRACTICE

Models

Understandings influencing current policy and practice in community care services in many countries for people with serious mental health problems and physical disability (Means & Smith 1999), are articulated in the WHO (1980) model of disability. This model defines the nature of the difficulties faced by the disabled person as follows:

- *Impairment*–the person experiences loss or abnormality in biological or psychological functioning.
- *Disability*–the person is unable through impairment to carry out social roles.

- *Disadvantage*–through inability to carry out social roles the person suffers social disadvantage.

In this model, the roots of the difficulties experienced by disabled people continue to be thought to lie in impairments or abnormalities in biological and psychological functioning, and in the case of psychosis, those impairments are thought to involve disorders in the biological or psychological processes making 'reason' possible-i.e., in the disease of mental illness (Bracken & Thomas 2001), or in 'irrational' cognitions (Fowler 1998). These abnormalities or deficiencies of 'reason' are then thought to affect social functioning, in turn leading to social disadvantage. As Harris (1999) points out, 'even today, pure reason . . . is valued in popular culture as the proper basis for social, economic, and political relations, almost as much as it was in the Enlightenment' (Harris, 1999, p. 14), and this means people thought to lack this capacity of 'reason,' viewed as essential to human functioning (Stainton 2002), are as likely today as in the Enlightenment to be deemed unfit to participate in society.

Both historically and today, therefore, the key to mental health disability and social exclusion is thought to lie in 'deficiencies' (Williams 1996) in the person's *functioning*. What, then, does this focus on individual functioning as the basis of disability and social exclusion mean for policy and practice?

Policy Framework

Mental health community care policy in many industrialised countries in the second half of the 20th century did involve state-funded professional provision of both health and social care services, but by the 1990s many states had lessened their involvement in areas of social care provision, which had up to then, been regarded as 'essential welfare provision' (Prior 1999, p. 110). A big distinction was drawn (Goodwin 1997), still underpinning current policy, between 'therapeutic interventions, and the supportive care that is required for daily living' (Conway et al., 1996, p. 158).

Within this distinction treatment is understood to involve state-funded, skilled medical, psychological, and nursing interventions that only professionals can carry out, these having a direct impact on the biological or psychological 'impairments' of reasoning and problem-solving, with the aim of reducing the person's disability and through this, her/his welfare problems linked to social exclusion. Current policy thinking, however, has led to a new approach–albeit reminiscent of nineteenth century 'residual' policies (Spicker 1995) linked to the Enlightenment beliefs: This is the New Deal in the UK and similar policies in the USA (Nikolas & Peck 1999), and other western countries (Hyde 2000), which seek to reduce both disability and social exclusion amongst physically disabled people and people with serious mental health problems, by 'welfare to work' (Roulstone 2000). This involves providing opportunities in mainstream life to improve skills and motivation sufficiently to enable the person to obtain employment. This approach represents a radical departure from expert interventions with the person as a more passive object of treatment, but significantly it retains the focus of intervening with 'reason' and problem solving, as a means of reducing both disability and social exclusion.

Social care, on the other hand, aims to provide for needs such as practical and social care, accommodation, finance, education, employment, leisure, transport, and access (Great Britain: Department of Health/Social Services Inspectorate 1991, pp. 12-13). These can be seen to relate to social exclusion, and in contrast to therapeutic interventions with individual functioning, policy is likely to emphasise informal, non-professional, sources of assistance with these needs: UK policy, for example, recommends that 'most care will be carried out by family friends and neighbours, . . . and it is right' (Great Britain: Department of Health 1989, p. 4), and failing this, by unqualified staff in the private sector–in many countries paid for by private insurance (Goodwin 1997).

The Divide Between 'Reason' and 'Nature' in Policy

Treatment and Intervention

Treatment has its origins in ideas following from the Enlightenment and Darwin, that professionals–starting with doctors in the nineteenth century, but expanding to include psychologists, nurses, and social workers in the early 20th century (Barnes & Bowl 2001)–were scientists, using expert knowledge ('reason') to solve individuals' health and welfare problems.

With the rise of professionals, the causes of these problems were located entirely within the individual's poor functioning: The difficult circumstances s(he) was likely to be experiencing were seen as the result of the problems within her or him, rather than as making any contribution to their cause–thus 'social disorganisation' in the person's circumstances was viewed as the 'outward visible sign of moral and intellectual disorganisation' (Bosanquet 1901, 297, cited in Jones 1998, p. 43). Diagnosed thus as an inadequately functioning person, then, the individual with serious mental health problems was deemed closer to 'nature' than a human being, and hence professionals represented 'reason controlling nature' (Brandon 1991). Today these assumptions about the cause of serious mental health problems can be seen still in the relationship between mental health professionals, and service users: Professionals' continuing statutory powers over users, resembling those of a parent over a child, along with stigmatising attitudes, together form an impermeable 'divide' between these two groups (Wilson & Beresford 2000).

At the heart of this relationship today is the information processing concept of the stress vulnerability model of schizophrenia, currently highly influential (Taylor & Liberzon 1999). In this model, the individual is believed to have biological and psychological 'vulnerability factors' involving 'information processing deficits, autonomic reactivity anomalies and social competence and coping limitations' (Neuchterlein & Dawson 1984, p. 300). When faced with social stressors–'life events' and ongoing 'social and environmental stress'–the individual is thus unable to cope, biologically and psychologically, and this results in biochemical reactions which 'produce psychotic episodes' (Neuchterlein and Dawson 1984, p. 300). Cognitive behavioural therapy, as the currently most prominent form of psychological intervention with psychosis (Great Britain: Department of Health 1999a), similarly understands the problems of psychosis as significantly influenced by maladaptive perceptions and cognitions in respect of stressors (e.g., Fowler 1998).

In this model, then, although social stressors play a part in psychosis, they are thought to have an effect only through the person's poor biological and psychological functioning: the situation would be quite different with an ordinarily functioning person, expected to be able to 'resist stress' (Jahoda 1958), through adequate powers of 'reason.' And even the existence of stressors in the life of the person with serious mental health problems may be understood, in accord with the World Health Organisation (1980) model, as result of the person's history of poor mental functioning (Neuchterlein & Dawson 1984). 'Welfare to Work' similarly sees social exclusion ultimately as due to the person's failure of 'health and work readiness,' which is *not* an 'inevitable consequence of their condition' (Great Britain: Department of Social Security 1998), and thus targets these motivations and capacities with training, information, and personal advisors (Roulstone 2000).

Treatment and 'welfare to work,' therefore, as society's best attempt to reduce and, where possible, remove the person's experiences both of disability and of social exclusion, concern themselves with the person's functioning, rather than intervening with stressors themselves: on the contrary social care or support with stressors can often be seen as working against the person maximising her/his functioning–e.g., the threat of benefit *loss* is expected under New Deal policies (Nikolas & Peck 1999; Roulstone 2000) to keep the person attending programmes, and professionals have been found in one large survey to refer service users with serious mental health problems and high support needs, to near-independent tendencies, so as to encourage their independence (Audit Commission 1998).

Social Care

Social care has been defined by Bulmer (1987) as:

- Physical assistance
- Practical, financial, and emotional support and assistance
- Concern about the person's welfare

This can be understood as dealing with 'nature' aspects of the person–her/his body, environment, and emotions. These form the context, the circumstances in which the person seeks to function. It is these which constitute the person's experiences of social exclusion. As we have seen, however, it is not these experiences but the person's biological and psychological functioning, which is seen in both physical and mental health contexts, to make such a difference to disability–and ultimately to these very experiences of social exclusion. Thus professional commentators, besides policy-makers, delegate social care work in mental health to non-professional staff–'non-specific support, practical help or . . . access to ordinary social activities . . . are tasks which are all probably better done by untrained staff, working alongside professionals . . .' (Shepherd 1998, p. 174).

Intervention with these experiences, then, in terms of providing care, is regarded essentially as 'ordinary' (Finlay 2000, p. 91) i.e., as meeting needs, addressing the person's state of existence (on a parallel, perhaps, to feeding animals) in contrast to the technical, problem-solving skills involved in 'treatment,' believed necessary in Enlightenment thought to 'manipulate' (Scull 1983) the complex machinery intrinsic to the person's functioning.

Thus the provision of treatment and care seems to be viewed in terms of the contrast between 'reason' and 'nature,' with only the former thought to have the power to make improvements in mental health.

Social Work and the Divide

Mental health professionals seeking status and effectiveness within this set of societal understandings, therefore, consider their role should primarily involve attention to the person's functioning, choosing as its major focus:

- Treatment and symptoms
- Motivation for treatment

- Monitoring mental state and behaviour
- Poor relationship and coping skills

(Shepherd 1995; Pepper & Perkins 1995)

Social care work on the other hand has been downgraded historically (Davis 1985) and today:

- Community support staff (unqualified staff helping with social care needs in the community) have been seen as doing 'hands on' work by mental health professionals, who saw themselves in contrast as working 'professionally' (Murray et al., 1998).
- Social workers have been described by health staff in relation to their social care work as 'untrained,' 'not professional,' 'undisciplined' (Higgins 1999, p. 273).

However, social workers tend to share these perceptions of social care with health professionals (Higgins 1999), demonstrating concerns, equal to those of the latter, with trying to address the person's functioning as a means of meeting needs (Worth 2002).

Historically, precursors of today's social workers in the charity organisation society in the UK and its parallels in the USA and elsewhere had as their 'principal concern either the moral education of clients, or their supervision. Material circumstances were considered largely as an external measure of personal and familial morality' (Jones 1998, p. 36). Thus even though their remit was to intervene with social care problems, they shared the wider professional and societal understandings about their origin and the need for intervention in the person's (moral) functioning. And although social work today would not concern itself with morality, a focus on coping–and therefore functioning–prevails: mental health social workers a few years ago exhorted users to 'face their problems' (Mitchell 1993); provided teaching or counselling as the sole or primary intervention in all but 5% of cases (Sheppard 1991), and today are often concerned with cognitive therapy (Norman & Peck 1999)–clearly focused on 'reason' itself, and primarily concerned with problem-solving (Howe 1997)–and skills training (Milner & O'Brien 2000).

At the same time, however, social work values of anti-discriminatory practice (Thompson 2001), aspire to counter the types of stigma, discrimination and disempowerment that can follow from the functioning-oriented 'treatment' approach (Wilson & Beresford 2000). But from these perspectives too, the focus in work with individuals is on functioning, through a concern with enabling them to maximise their control over their lives (Thompson 1998; Dalrymple & Burke 1995). Thus cognitive therapy can again be a favoured individual intervention–albeit from a more radical perspective (Corob

1987); solution-focussed therapy involving narrative has been proposed (Milner 2002), and practitioners taking a feminist perspective have understood depressed women to need help with internalised self-limiting beliefs about themselves resulting from gender discrimination in society (Crocker & Shephard 1999). Howe (1997) has pointed out that problem-solving cognitive explanations and interventions with problems tend to leave emotions out of the picture–and this will be so regardless of whether their orientation is radical or traditional–and Crocker and Shephard (1999) similarly observe that these practitioners' understandings served to 'minimise the degree of emotional trauma suffered' (1999, p. 603). Material and practical help also forms no part of these approaches.

Overall, then, both health and social care professionals have concerns reflecting the Enlightenment divide between 'reason' and 'emotion,' 'mind' and 'nature,' seeking to maximise the person's mental health and independent functioning by working on the 'reason' side of the divide, i.e., the person's biological functioning and psychological coping–while relegating 'emotion' and 'nature' to the 'hands on' work of unqualified staff. This is not to say that interventions with functioning are of no value, but rather to turn a light on to the care side of the divide: It has been dismissed to the farthest shadows, but its reality is perhaps at the opposite extreme, with the potential to turn mental health interventions right around.

Alternative Perspective

There are important critiques of this legacy of the Enlightenment in mental health (Bracken & Thomas 2001), and in other areas such as employment (Nikolas & Peck 1999), and offending, as expressed by the comment that 'stress on offending behaviour entails the expectation that offenders and not their social circumstances must change, and encourages the abstraction of the offending act itself from the (social) context which would make it intelligible' (Smith 1998, p. 108 cited in Barry 2000, p. 589).

A recent development in sociology is the social realist perspective, which has the potential to take us further into this perspective in mental health. From the Enlightenment perspective, individual 'reason'–or mental capacity–is seen as the dominant force, making for good or poor social functioning–but the realist position suggests that emotion, environment and the body, deemed as of little significance in the latter, in fact, play the major role. This view is found in parts of the social work literature–Howe (1997) for example suggests that the emotions arising from social stressors form the basis for poor social functioning, and Bywaters and McLeod (1996) point out that disadvantaged environments are 'lived out physically and psychologically' (Bywaters & McLeod 1996, p. 16).

The realist position draws on research in the physical health context to suggest that social conditions and the emotional response to these can play a major role in the production of physical diseases. Hence 'the emotionally expressive body translates broader psychosocial and material conditions of existence into the recalcitrant language of disease and disorder' (Williams 1998, p. 64).

Let us consider, then, where this perspective can take us in respect of the relationship between social exclusion and psychosis.

Social Exclusion and Mental Health

What is social exclusion? We can understand it as exclusion from mainstream social life, taking place within the two dimensions of society traditionally conceptualised by sociologists (Becker 1997). These include

- Structure–denial of resources and opportunities–e.g., in employment, housing, income, education
- Culture–devaluing attitudes, beliefs, and actions–e.g., racist stereotypes, abuse of any sort, following from perceptions of the victim as inferior (Aitken 1996).

Many critics (e.g., Sayce 2000; Dunn 1999; Pilgrim 1997) of biological and individual models of mental health problems point to statistics linking aspects of social exclusion to mental health problems, and social inclusion to recovery, suggesting that it is social exclusion rather than individual 'deficiencies' that are disabling. Social realism has much to say on the processes by which this may take place.

As a basis for considering these processes–i.e., how exclusion may work through the 'emotionally expressive body' (Williams 1998) to play a part in psychosis–let us first explore some aspects of social exclusion experienced by people with long-term psychoses.

Looking first at how far social exclusion may be implicated in the onset of psychosis, we will need to consider experiences of the former which precede the latter. Research findings on social exclusion preceding psychosis include the following:

- People originating in lower socio-economic groups experience serious mental health problems longer term, and have higher rates of relapse, than people from higher socio-economic groups (Thornicroft 1993).

- People developing long term serious mental health problems experience prior disadvantage–poverty, poor housing, isolation, poor education, few life skills–at high rates (Castle et al., 1993).
- People with mental health problems have significantly higher rates of unemployment prior to developing these problems than people in the population not developing these problems (Melzer et al., 1995).
- People with serious mental health problems will have experienced childhood physical and sexual abuse at twice the rate of the general population (Read 1997).

Second we can consider ongoing experiences of social exclusion faced by those with long-term serious mental health problems:

- This group experiences poverty and disadvantage at 2-3 times the rate of the general population (Henderson et al., 1998).
- Up to 85% are unemployed (Bird 1999).
- Homelessness–7% in inner cities (Johnson 1997).
- 47% verbally or physically harassed in public (Read & Baker 1996).
- 90% felt people feared them (Rose 1996).

Third, in relation to recovery, comparative findings across different types of society also show a striking link to social exclusion–65% of people with schizophrenia recover in traditional societies where they are accepted and participate to the extent they can manage in social roles, in contrast with only 28% in western and industrial societies where they are rejected and excluded from social roles (Warner 1994).

EMOTION AND BIOLOGY

Realist Perspective

We have seen that the stress vulnerability model of serious mental health problems, while acknowledging stress, locates the essential cause of psychosis in abnormal mental functioning. How can the realist approach relate to this?

In fact research has shown that emotions are implicated in the process thought to lead through this model to psychosis. Reactivity itself, associated with psychotic symptoms in the model (Neuchterlein & Dawson 1984, Warner 1994), is an emotional response of anxiety, manifesting itself in high levels of central nervous system arousal, and emotions of anxiety and depression are present immediately before relapse in a majority of people diagnosed with schizophrenia (Hirsch 1991).

However, in most understandings of human response currently accepted, emotions are viewed simply as the products of other ultimately intra-individual processes–e.g., the individual's biology or her/his internalised social beliefs (Williams 1998, pp. 56-57)–and in the stress vulnerability model similarly, the above emotions are seen as the result of the person's poor biological or psychological functioning in relation to stress (Birchwood 1993): they are therefore viewed as having only a minimal connection to actual stressors.

The realist position, however, argues that emotions usually are not so 'irrational,' but form 'realistic assessments and understandable responses to extreme social circumstances' (Williams 1998, p. 65), and as such can be linked to physical disease: For example, the work of Marmot et al. (1991) shows the emotions linked to unemployment and job insecurity have an impact on endocrinal and immunological biological disorders associated with heart disease, cancer, and other diseases. Can such links be so with mental ill-health?

Recent research (Pitman 1997) suggests that it can. One aspect of social exclusion experienced by as many as 60-70% of people with psychoses (Read 1997) is that of abuse. Research into the psychobiological impact of trauma shows that post traumatic stress, thought previously to have a psychological effect only, affects biological processes leading to both physical and mental health problems. And in accord with the realist position above showing it is *extreme* emotions that can link up to biology in this way to form physical disease, so trauma too involves persistent and extreme emotions.

Let us return then to the stressors faced by people developing long term psychosis. How extreme are they?

'The most striking characteristic of the study sample were just how poor living standards and quality of life were overall, and second by just how inadequately current models of care addressed these deficits.' (Firth & Bridges 1999, p. 135)

'Poverty itself can contribute to ill health. Money worries together with the circumstances that cause them–job loss, onset of ill health, relationship breakdown–can lead to . . . anxiety and depression.' (Walker & Walker 1998, p. 52)

Abuse involves *'shattering'* of the person's *'sense of personal invulnerability to harm,' 'perception of the world as meaningful,' 'positive feelings about the self.'* (Patten 1989, p. 199),

'I'm ashamed of living where I am and that makes me feel depressed.'
(Barham & Hayward 1991, p. 52)

Undoubtedly these are extreme experiences, and research on the effects of trauma shows that extreme emotions can be specifically linked to psychotic symptoms. Although only about 1% of most populations are diagnosed with schizophrenia (Warner 1994), and in community surveys about 2% at any one time experience hallucinations (Tien 1991)–a central psychotic symptom–as many as 64% of people who had experienced childhood sexual abuse experienced these symptoms (Chu & Dill 1990), and Ensink (1993) confirms that such experiences are identical to those diagnosed as symptoms of schizophrenia.

It is also important to note the connection between 'anxiety and depression' as a result of the above social stressors, and these emotions as precursors of psychosis. The indication in the above research findings that the stressors involved in social exclusion are so severe that people experiencing them have *every* reason, rather than 'no reason to feel as they do' (Crossley 2000, p. 280), suggests that the presence of these emotions prior to psychosis may be less 'unreasonable,' less a product of abnormal mental functioning, than has been thought. And research findings discussed by Goldberg and Huxley (1992) that as many as 70% of the general population may experience 'common mental disorders' in disadvantaged areas lends strong support to this view.

A Social Solution?

It, therefore, appears that psychotic symptoms have links to real emotions, arising in response to experiences of social exclusion, i.e., psychotic symptoms appear at a high rate amongst people who have experienced abuse, and the precursors of psychosis are common responses to extreme social stressors. This suggests the important possibility, parallel to findings in the areas of physical disease and trauma, that the emotions commonly connected to social stressors may also play a role in the biological processes underpinning psychosis and some evidence for this is summarised by Warner (2000, p. 31).

What might this mean for mental health interventions? In the physical health context, regarding the commonly experienced effects of social stressors as important in the generation of biological disease carries implications for policies and practices that aim to reduce social inequalities (Duggan 2002), and the statistical links of mental ill-health to social exclusion have similarly led to calls for a primarily 'social solution' to psychosis (Repper & Perkins 1996).

However, this cannot be the only solution. This is because many people exposed to extreme stressors do not develop psychosis, i.e., two thirds experiencing trauma do not develop post traumatic stress (Rose 1994), let alone associated psychotic symptoms. This is not incompatible with the belief of the stress vulnerability model that there are innate differences in 'reactivity,' but this is a belief inimical to anti-discriminatory social work values: the possibility of innate reactivity, as we have seen, has meant historically and currently that the person is 'deficient'–falls short of the Enlightenment expectation of a human being as able to 'resist stress'–and this has resulted in the person being denied rights and stigmatised.

These attitudes originate, however, with the Enlightenment and Darwin, as values and beliefs attached to 'reason.' 'Emotion' and the body, where the person profoundly affected by strong emotions and biological reactions is seen as 'backward' (Furnham & Rees 1992)–still under the sway of 'archaic remnants' that people who are fully human, can master. If instead we recognise that it is only from the above historical–and Eurocentric (Lago & Thompson 1996)–perspectives, that being affected emotionally is seen as inferior, we may start to view 'reactivity' differently, i.e., as 'valued difference,' as Morris (1991) suggests in relation to the physical 'impairments' underlying physical disability.

Of significance here would be the physical diseases of asthma and heart disease. Medical understandings of these conditions suggest there to be predispositional factors operating on the same way as reactivity with psychosis, and medical interventions work in the same way as medication with schizophrenia in relation to these factors: the role of medication in both cases is to reduce the physiological response to stress–to act as a protective 'buffer' (Hirsch 1991). However, in these physical ill-health examples, crucially, the person is not seen as any less of a person because of her/his 'predispositions'–this is because they do not represent deviations from what is considered to be 'human.'

The suggests, therefore, that reactivity can be seen aside from Enlightenment values, as similar simply to the biological variants operating generally in physical ill-health, and if we further take into account the important findings from psychobiological research into trauma, we can arrive at the following understandings of the role of reactivity in psychosis:

- As a response to real emotions arising from real circumstances that are extremely stress-provoking.
- As an emotional response rather than a product of a perhaps irremediable 'deficiency' of functioning.
- As a human variant with no connotations of inferiority–some people react more to emotions than others.

These understandings change our perspective: the person is no longer sub-human, lacking what it takes to function as a human being. Instead s(he) is a 'person in situation'–someone affected by and responding to her/his social circumstances as a human being, in ways characteristic of her/him. But the extreme and traumatic nature of these circumstances will mean the person's responses involve pain and disturbance.

Emotions and Psychosis

The preceding suggests, therefore, that the emotional impact of extreme social adversity and exclusion may have an influence in its own right upon biology: an impact that can lead to psychosis in more sensitive individuals. This calls into question the weight placed, in current and historical belief, upon individual mental functioning as the crucial factor in the process leading to psychosis, and if it is correct, it has significant implications for practice.

Within this perspective, these emotional and biological effects of adversity have consequences for the person's functioning and therefore both this and the functioning perspective have a concern with addressing the latter. However, in accord with Howe's (1987) point that our explanations are what make the difference to our practices, if we take the functioning perspective, then the person's capacities will be the focus of intervention, but if the explanation focuses more on the effects of the person's experiences, the pain undergone, then intervention will be primarily concerned with relief of that pain, whether biological, psychological, or social.

Indications that this approach may have validity are found in repeated research findings that social care has the power not only to elicit user satisfaction, but to improve mental health outcomes. In one study (Shephard 1991), people with mental health problems found the relationship of empathy, understanding, and concern for them more helpful to their mental health than any treatment intervention, and in different studies, users found the same client-centred, concerned relationship with their care manager, along with committed attempts to help with practical problems and family tensions 'helped keep me out of hospital' and be 'more independent' (Ryan et al., 1999, Beeforth et al., 1994), thus reducing relapse and improving social functioning. Murray et al., (1998) also report that 87% and 75% of users respectively in their sample found emotional support and help with practical difficulties the 'most helpful' interventions. These findings thus demonstrate connections between service users' social care needs, and mental health and social functioning outcomes.

At the same time, research with service users has shown up that medical interventions are also valued as important (Shepherd 1995; Ferguson 1997)–what users in these studies found particularly unhelpful in this connection was the devaluing relationship (Ferguson 1997) in which they are made to feel inferior (as indeed they are perceived to be, on the basis of the historical beliefs about mental ill-health discussed earlier). Of significance here is the point that users value medication when it relieves symptoms and distress (Mental Health Foundation 1997), and this again is about an experience of *care*.

MODELS FOR PRACTICE

These understandings suggest, therefore, that the model of a biologically and emotionally 'embodied' (Williams 1998) 'person in situation' may form a meaningful basis for mental health social work practice with psychosis. These understandings do relate to existing 'biopsychosocial' models (Onyett 1992), and their recent developments (Coppock & Hopton 2000), but carry particular practice implications that contrast with the 'functioning' perspective so widely informing current mental health interventions.

In this model workers would

- Work alongside biological interventions
- Practice psychological interventions
- Practice social interventions

They would do this within an egalitarian, respecting relationship rather than through the current 'divide' (Wilson & Beresford 2000), because service users are recognised as people experiencing the effects of lived experiences, rather than as sub human creatures 'deficient' (Williams 1996) in their functioning. This way of seeing mental health problems also means interventions have more focus on care–providing healing and relief from pain affecting the person biologically, psychologically, and socially: People are perceived as having a *right* to concern, supports, resources, promoting their well-being, in contrast to the sociohistorical beliefs about service users from 'deficiency' models, described earlier.

Within this model, functioning interventions would still be important–e.g., Corney and Clare (1983) shows how women with severe depression undertook day-to-day tasks they could manage, and achievement of these had benefits for self-esteem, contributing, along with social, practical, and emotional support, to reduction in depression. Also more disabled people with psychosis have never had the opportunity to develop life skills, and service users provided with these opportunities in a hostel ward (Reid & Garety 1996) experienced more well-being, better functioning, and accessed more independent living arrangements. Thus there are many occasions where functioning interventions can also address the effects and biopsychosocial adversity upon the person and her/his life. However, by placing these within a context that recognises functioning difficulties not as deficiency, but as the effects of extreme adversity on a person, with all that this means for attitudes and responses, the person is not demeaned, and is offered sufficient of the range of supports s(he) needs alongside direct help with functioning, with the overall valuing and restorative aim of offering healing.

Rethinking Interventions

Biological Interventions

Anti-discriminatory values in social work have led to a particular rejection of psychiatry and biological interventions as the source of stigma in the mental health context (Thompson 1998) through their appearing to signify a fundamental deficiency in the person's make-up. But the stigma here comes from the wider societal constructs of mental ill-health, whether understood biologically, psychologically or morally, as a deficiency of personhood. This suggests that different understandings about biology in mental health can remove the stigma of these interventions and thus enable working relationships with psychiatrists to be transformed.

Thus if biological disturbance in mental ill health is understood as a result of being particularly affected by extreme experiences, the experiences of suffering–feeling both mentally and physically ill (Kendall 2001)–can be more recognised, and medication as care can come into play, enabling the person to feel better, and consequently to cope better–just as with physical illness.

However, the worker is also in a position, with a developed appreciation of the role of medical interventions, to challenge prescribing that is unhelpful, producing effects that do not enable the person to feel better and cope better (Mental Health Foundation 1997).

Psychological Interventions

There is much focus on an 'educative' approach today (Harrison et al., 1996), in which psychological interventions such as cognitive therapy that teach coping, are given significance with psychoses (Conway et al., 1996). There is a place for these, valued by some service users (e.g., Hardy et al., 1998) but what may be called the 'social care' form of counselling, focusing on concern–which as we saw earlier is another component of social care–also has a place.

This would involve person-centred counselling, enabling the person to find relief from emotional pain in a warm, understanding, non-judgmental relationship with the worker (Hughes & Hughes 1998). By relieving pain, this approach has the power to enable the individual to become 'more able to think, and eventually to make sense of feelings and experiences which have previously been felt to be overwhelming' (Hughes & Hughes 1998, p. 72). Thus predominantly non-verbal help here has the potential to increase mental functioning, and through that, the person's degree of control over her/his life.

Social Interventions

Empowering social care interventions have often been seen in terms of helping the person to better control her/his own life: The aims of the empowering social care relationship have been seen to include the following: 'to build capacity, to equip people with personal resources of self-esteem and confidence, and to share knowledge and skills (Braye 2000, p. 21). However, the importance of egalitarian social care, involving the worker in providing resources, support and practical assistance, as we have seen, plays a crucial role in empowerment addressing difficulties the person is, or feels, unable to cope with, through the effects of biopsychosocial adversity. This is the 'social component' of Bulmer's (1987) definition of social care.

This is not the unskilled work it is thought by professionals (Higgins 1999) to be: For example, for the many users with serious mental health problems who are unable to cope with independent tendencies (Audit Commission 1998), the stress of this, and possible eviction, is likely to lead to relapse and exacerbated social adversity and risk through becoming homeless (Lipscombe 1997). A lot of skills are involved in conducting an accurate assessment of these housing and support needs–and indeed the range of social care needs–in partnership with the service user, as also in being able to negotiate appropriate resources to meet the needs (Murray et al., 1998), and this will make all the difference to whether the person can cope and feel better, or relapse and risk losing everything.

At the same time, the advantages of functioning interventions in improving well-being and the person's freedom to live the life s(he) wants, must not be forgotten. As Braye and Preston-Shoot (1995) point out, it is disempowering to over- or under-provide either supports or direct capacity building interventions in relation to what the person feels able to cope with, and what s(he) aspires to–e.g., more supports that the person feels they need can lead her/him to feel inferior. Again, skilled assessment in full partnership with the service user is essential in ensuring this balance is right for her/him, and if this is carried out within the fundamental approach of egalitarian care in relation to adversity, rather than that of acting on a 'deficient' being, the person is experiencing responsiveness and respect in every aspect of the intervention and the worker's attitudes, and this provides holistic conditions in which the person can experience greater well-being, through reduction in the impacts of biopsychosocial adversity upon her/his social care concerns, thus becoming freer to live the life s(he) wants.

CONCLUSIONS

We have considered in this article how psychosis can be seen in a different way from that currently influential, and some of the implications such a change in perspective may have on practice.

Psychosis has been seen as a deficiency in biological and psychological functioning, but research on the psychobiological reactions to of extreme social conditions can lead to a different view, in which psychotic symptoms are seen more as results of the emotional and biological effects of social adversity upon individuals who are particularly sensitive.

The emphasis on suffering and distress in this model carries practice implications for a greater emphasis on providing care in a valuing relationship, in order to relieve pain and stress, and this is to provide a direct response to the 'person in situation'–her/his circumstances, resulting emotions, and ultimately her/his biology and psychotic symptoms. Through this, there is evidence that symptoms can reduce, and the person's health and social functioning can improve.

There is also a new respect overcoming the traditional worker-user 'divide' (Wilson & Beresford 2000) inherent in this intervention approach, as there is no assumption that workers are perfected 'reason' controlling a deficient 'nature'; rather, they are working in partnership with another human being to maximise her/his experience of well-being and through this to enable her/him to increase control over her/his life.

REFERENCES

Aitken, L. (1996). Gender issues in elder abuse. London: Sage.

Audit Commission for Local Authorities & the National Health Service in England & Wales. (1998). Home alone: The role of housing in community care. London: Audit Commission.

Barham, P., & Hayward, R. (1991). From the mental patient to the person. London: Routledge.

Barnes, M., & Bowl, R. (2001). Taking over the asylum: Empowerment and mental health. Basingstoke: Palgrave.

Barry, M. (2000). The Mentor-Monitor debate in criminal justice–'what works' for offenders. *British Journal of Social Work.* 30 (5), 575-597.

Becker, S. (1997). Responding to poverty. London: Longman.

Beeforth, M., Conlan, E., & Grayley, R. (1994). Have we got views for you: User evaluation of case management. London: Sainsbury Centre for Mental Health.

Bentall, R. (1990). Syndromes and symptoms of schizophrenia. In R. Bentall (ed.), Reconstructing schizophrenia. (pp. 23-59). London: Routledge.

Birchwood, M. (1993). Depression, demoralisation, and control over psychotic illness. Psychological medicine. 23 (2), 387-395.

Bird, L. (1999). The fundamental facts–all the latest facts and figures on mental illness: Mental Health Foundation.

Bosanquet, B. (1901). The meaning of social work. *International Journal of Ethics.* 11, 297.

Bracken, P., & Thomas, P. (2001). Post psychiatry: A new direction for mental health. British Medical Journal. 322, 724-727.

Brandon, D. (1991). Innovation without change: Consumer power in psychiatric services. Basingstoke, Macmillan.

Braye, S. (2000). Participation and involvement in social care. In H. Kemshall & R. Littlechild (eds.), User involvement and participation in social care. (pp. 9-28). London: Jessica Kingsley.

Braye, S., & Preston Shoot, M. (1995). Empowering practice in social care. Buckingham, Open University Press.

Bulmer, M. (1987). The social basis of community care. London: Allen & Unwin.

Bywaters, P., & McLeod, E. (1996). Working for equality in health. London: Routledge.

Carmen, J. (1984). Victims of Violence and Psychiatric Illness. *American Journal of Psychiatry.* 141, 378-383.

Castle, D., Scott, K., Wessely, S., & Murray, R. (1993). Does social deprivation during gestation and early life predispose to schizophrenia? Social Psychiatry and Psychiatric Epidemology. 28, 1-4.

Chu, J.A., & Dill, D.L. (1990). Dissociative symptoms in relation to childhood physical and sexual abuse. *American Journal of Psychiatry.* 147. 887-892.

Conway, M., Shepherd, G., & Melzer, D. (1996). Effectiveness of interventions for mental illness and implications for commissioning. In G. Strathdee, & G. Thornicroft (eds.), Commissioning mental health services. London: HMSO.

Coppock, V., & Hopton, J. (2000). Critical Perspectives on Mental Health. London: Routledge.

Corney, R., & Clare, A. (1983). The effectiveness of attached social workers in the management of depressed women in general practice. *British Journal of Social Work.* 13, 57-74.

Crocker, G., & Sheppard, M. (1999). The psychosocial 'diagnosis' of depression in mothers: An exploration and analysis. *British Journal of Social Work.* 29, 601-620.

Crossley, N. (2000). Emotions, psychiatry, and social order: A Habermasian approach. In S. Williams, J. Gabe & M. Calnan (eds.), Health, medicine, and society: Key theories/future agendas. (pp. 277-295). London: Routledge.

Cuff, E.C. (2000). Perspectives in sociology, Fifth Edition. London: Unman Hyman.

Dalley, G. (1988). Ideologies of caring. Basingstoke, UK: Macmillan.

Dalyrmple, J., & Burke, B. (1995). Anti-oppressive practice, social care, and the law. Buckingham, UK: Open University Press.

Davey, B. (1994). Mental health and the environment: Care in place. *International Journal of Networks and Community. 1* (2), 118-201.

Duggan, M. (2002). Social exclusion and health promotion. In L. Adams, M. Amos, & J. Munro (eds), Promoting health: Policies and practices. London, Thousand Oaks, New Delhi: Sage.

Dunn, S. (1999). Creating accepting communities: Report of the Mind inquiry into social exclusion and mental health problem. London: MIND (National Association for Mental Health).

Ensink, B. (1993). Trauma: A study of childhood abuse and hallucinations. In M. Romme & S. Escher (eds.), Accepting voices. London: MIND Publications.

Ferguson, I. (1997). The Impact of Mental Health User Involvement. Research, Policy, and Planning. 15(2), 26-30.

Finlay, L. (2000). The challenge of professionalism. In A. Brechin, H. Brown, & M.A. Eby (eds.), Critical practice in health and social care (pp. 73-95). Buckingham UK and London: Sage and Open University Press.

Firth, M.T., & Bridges, K. (1996). Brief social work intervention for people with severe and persistent disorders. *Journal of Mental Health.* 5 (2), 135-143.

Fowler, D. et al. (1998). Cognitive therapy for psychosis: From treatment, effectiveness, and service implications. *Journal of Mental Health.* 7(2), 123-133.

Furnham, A., & Rees, J. (1988). Lay theories of schizophrenia. *The International Journal of Social Psychiatry.* 34 (3), 212-220.

Giddens, A (1998). The third way: The renewal of social democracy. Cambridge: Policy.

Goldberg, D., & Huxley, P. (1992). Common mental disorders. London: Tavistock/ Routledge.

Golding, P., & Middleton, S. (1982). Images of welfare. London: Martin Robertson.

Goodwin, S. (1997). Comparative mental health policy. London: Sage.

Gordon, D., Adelman, L., Ashworth, C., Bradshaw, J., Levitas, R., Middleton, S., Pantazis, C., Patsios, D., Payne, S., Townsend, P., & Williams, J. (2000). Poverty and Social Exclusion in Britain. York: Joseph Rowntree Foundation.

Great Britain: Department of Health (1999a). Mental Health: National Service Frameworks. London: Department of Health.

Great Britain: Department of Health (1999b). Saving lives. CM.4386. London: The Stationery Office.

Great Britain: Department of Health (2000). A quality strategy for social care. London: HMSO.

Great Britain: Department of Health (2001). Making it happen (Mental Health Promotions). London: Department of Health.

Great Britain: Department of Health. (1989). Caring for people: Community care in the next decade and beyond. London: HMSO.

Great Britain: Department of Health/Social Services Inspectorate. (1991). Practioners' guide to care management and assessment. London: HMSO.

Great Britain: Department of Social Security (1998). Harman introduces radical strategy for disabled people. Press release, 9th July, London: Department of Social Security.

Grove, B. (1998). Mental health and employment: Shaping a new agenda. *Journal of Mental Health.* 7 (2), 131-140.

Hardy, G.E., Shapiro, D.A., Stiles, W.B., & Barkham, M. (1998). When and why does cognitive behavioural treatment appear more effective than psychodynamic-interpersonal treatment? Discussion of the findings from the Second Sheffield Psychotherapy Project. *Journal of Mental Health.* 7 (2), 179-190.

Harris, R. (1999). Mental disorder and social order. In D. Webb & R. Harris (eds.), Mentally disordered offenders: Managing people nobody owns. (pp. 10-26). London: Routledge.

Harrison, C., Davies, P., & Pietroni, P. (1996). A controlled trial of self-care classes in general practice. In P. Pietroni & L. Petrioni (eds.), Innovation in community care and primary health. New York: Churchill Liningstone.

Henderson, C., Thornicroft, G., & Glover, G. (1998). Inequalities in mental health. *British Journal of Psychiatry.* 173, 105-109.

Higgins, R. (1994). Working together. Health and Social Care in the Community. 2, 269-277.

Hirsch, S. (1991). Maintenance medication for schizophrenia. In P.E. Bebbington (ed.), Social Psychiatry. (pp. 389-399). London: Transaction Publishers.

Howe, D. (1987). An introduction to social work theory. Aldershot, UK: Wildwood House.

Howe, D. (1997). Relating theory to practice. In M. Davies (ed.), The Blackwell companion to social work. (pp. 170-176). Oxford, UK: Blackwell.

Hughes, J., & Hughes, N. (1998). Therapeutic responses to people with learning disabilities who have been abused. In S. Bear (ed.), Good practice in counselling people who have been abused. (pp. 65-78). London: Jessica Kingsley.

Hyde, M. (2000). From Welfare to Work: Social policy for disabled people of working age in the United Kingdom in the 1990s. Disability and Society (2), 327-341.

Ingleby, D. (1983). Mental health and social order. In S. Cohen and A. Scull (eds.), Social Control and the State. (pp. 141-188). London: Martin Robertson.

Jahoda, M. (1958). Current conceptions of positive mental health. New York: Basic Books.

Johnson, S. (Ed.). (1997). London's mental health: The report for the Kings Fund London Commission. London: Kings Fund.

Jones, C. (1998). Social work and society. In R. Adams, L. Dominelli, & M. Payne (eds.), Social work: Themes, issues, and critical debates. (pp. 34-43). Basingstoke, UK: Macmillan.

Kendall, P. (2001). The distinction between mental and physical illness. *British Journal of Psychiatry.* 178 490-493

Lago, C., & Thompson, J. (1996) Race, culture and counseling. Buckingham, UK: Open University Press.

Lipscombe, S. (1997). Homelessness and mental health risk assessment. In H. Kemshall & J. Pritchard (eds.), Good practice in risk assessment and risk management. (pp. 141-158). London: Jessica Kingsley.

Macpherson, C.B. (1962). The political theory of possessive individualism. Oxford, UK: Oxford University Press.

Marmot, M., Smith, D., Stansfield, S., Patel, C., North, F., & Head, J. (1991). Health inequalities among British civil servants: The Whitehall II study. Lancet. 337, 1387-1393.

Melzer, H., Gil, B., Petticrew, M., & Hinds, K. (1995). The prevalence of psychiatric morbidity among adults living in private households. London: HMSO.

Mental Health Foundation (1997). Knowing our own minds. London: Mental Health Foundation.

Milner, J., & O'Brien, P. (2000). Assessment in Social Work. Basingstoke: Palgrave.

Milner, J. (2001). Women and Social Work–a narrative approach. Basingstoke: Palgrave.

Mitchell, R. (1993). Crisis intervention in practice: The multi-disciplinary team and mental health social work. Aldershot, Avebury: Macmillan.

Morris, J. (1991). Pride against prejudice. London: Women's Press.

Murray, A., Shepherd, G., & Onyett, S. (1997). More than a friend. London: The Sainsbury Centre for Mental Health.

Neuchterlein, K.H., & Dawson, M.E. (1984). A heuristic vulnerability/stress model of schizophrenic episodes. Schizophrenia Bulletin. 10 (2), 300-312.

Nicholas, T., & Peck, J. (1999). Welfare to work: National problems, local solutions? Critical Social Policy. 19 (4), 485-510.

Norman, I., & Peck, E. (1999). Working together in adult community mental health services: An inter professional dialogue. *Journal of Mental Health.* 8(3), 217-230.

O'Brien, M., & Penna, S. (1998). Theorising welfare. London: Sage.

Oliver, M. (1996). Understanding disability–from theory to practice. Basingstoke: Macmillan.

Onyett, S. (1992). Case management in mental health. London: Chapman and Hall.

Patten, S. B., Gatz, Y.K., Jones, B., & Thomas, D.L. (1989). Post-traumatic stress disorder and the treatment of sexual abuse. Social Work. May, 197-203.

Pilgrim, D. (1997). Some reflections on quality and mental health. *Journal of Mental Health.* 6 (6), 567-576.

Pitman, R.K. (1997). Overview of biological themes in PTSD. In R. Yehuda & A.C. McFarlane (eds.), Psychobiology of post-traumatic stress disorder. (pp. 1-9). New York: Annals of the New York Academy of Sciences, 821, June 21.

Prior, P. (1999). Gender and mental health. Basingstoke, UK.

Read, J. (1997). Child abuse and psychosis. Professional Psychology, Research, and Practice. 28 (5), 448-456.

Read, J., & Baker, S. (1996). Not just sticks and stones: A survey of the stigma, taboos, and discrimination experienced by people with mental health problems. London: MIND Publications.

Reid, Y. & Garety, P. (1996). A hostel-ward for new long stay patients: Sixteen years progress. *Journal of Mental Health.* 5(1), 77-90.

Repper, J., & Perkins, R. (1995). The deserving and the undeserving: Selectivity and progress in a community care service. *Journal of Mental Health.* 4 (5), 483-495.

Repper, J., & Perkins, R. (1996). Working alongside people with long-term mental health problems. Cheltenham, UK: Stuart-Thornes.

Ripa, Y. (1990). Women and Madness. Cambridge: Cambridge & Policy Press.

Rogers, A., & Pilgrim, D. (2001). Mental Health Policy in Britain (2nd ed). Basingstoke: Palgrave

Rose, D. (1996). In our experience. London: Sainsbury Centre for Mental Health.

Rose, S. (1994). Counselling following trauma. Counselling. May, 125-127.

Roth, A., & Fonagy, P. (1996). What works for whom? New York: Guilford Press.

Roulstone, A. (2000). Disability, dependency, and the New Deal for disabled people. Disability and Society. 15(3), 427-443.

Ryan, P., Ford, R., Bearsmoore, A., & Muijen, M. (1999). The enduring relevance of case management. *British Journal of Social Work.* 29 (1), 97-126.

Sayce, L. (1998). Stigma, discrimination, and social exclusion: what's in a word? *Journal of Mental Health.* 7 (4), 331-343.

Scull, A. (1983). Humanitarianism or control? In S. Cohen & A. Scull (eds.), Social control and the state. (pp. 118-140). London: Martin Robertson.

Shepherd, G. (1998). Models of community care. *Journal of Mental Health.* 7 (2), 165-77.

Shepherd, G., Murray, A., & Muijen, M. (1995). Perspectives on schizophrenia: A survey of user, family care, and professional views regarding effective care. *Journal of Mental Health. 4* (4), 403-422.

Sheppard, M. (1991). Mental health work in the community: Theory and practice in social work and community psychiatric nursing. London: Falmer Press.

Smith, D. (1998). Social work with offenders: The practice of exclusion & the policy for inclusion. In M. Barry & C. Hallett (eds.), Social exclusion and social work: issues of theory, policy and practice. Lyme Regis, UK: Russell House Publishers.

Social Services Inspectorate. (1999). Still building bridges. London: The Stationery Office.

Statham, D. (2000). Partnership between health and social care. Health and Social Care in the Community. 8 (2), 87-89.

Strathdee, G., & Thornicroft, G. (1996). Core components of a mental health service. In G. Strathdee & G. Thornicroft (eds.), Commissioning mental health services. (pp. 86-94). London: HMSO.

Taylor, S., & Liberzon, I. (1999). Paying attention to emotion in schizophrenia. *British Journal of Psychiatry.* 174, January, 6-8.

Thompson, N. (1998). Social work with adults. In R. Adams, L. Dominelli, & M. Payne (eds.), Social work: Themes, issues, and critical debates. (pp. 34-43). Basingstoke, UK: Macmillan.

Thompson, N. (2000a). Theory and practice in health and social care. In C. Davies, L. Finlay & A. Bullman (eds.), Changing practice in health and social care. London, Thousand Oaks, New Delhi: Sage.

Thompson, N. (2000b). Theory and practice in the human services (rev. ed) Buckingham: Open University Press.

Thompson, N. (2001). Anti-discriminatory practice (3rd ed.). Basingstoke, UK: Macmillan.

Thornicroft, G. (1993). Social deprivation and mental illness. *British Journal of Psychiatry.* 158, 475-484.

Tien, A.Y. (1991). Distribution of hallucinations in the population. Social Psychiatry & Psychiatric Epidemiology. 26, 287-292.

Walker, C., & Walker, A. (1998). Social policy and social work. In R. Adams, L. Dominelli & M. Payne (eds.), Social work: Themes, issues, and critical debates. (pp. 44-55). Basingstoke, UK: Macmillan.

Warner, R. (1994). Recovery from schizophrenia: Psychiatry and political economy (2nd ed.). London: Routledge.

Warner, R. (2000). The environment of schizophrenia: Innovations in practice, policies, and communities. London & Philadelphia: Brunner Routledge.

Williams, F. (1996). Race, welfare and community care: A historical perspective. In W. Ahmad & K. Atkins (eds.), Race and community care. (pp. 15-28). Buckingham: Open University Press.

Williams, J. (1998). Emotions, equity, and health. In A. Petersen, & C. Waddell (eds.), Health matters–a sociology of illness, prevention, and care. (pp. 55-71). Buckingham: Open University Press.

Wilson, A., Beresford, P. (2000). Surviving an abusive system. In H. Payne & B. Littlechild (eds.), Ethical practice and the abuse of power in social responsibility. (pp. 145-174). London: Kingsley.

World Health Organisation (1955). Hospitalisation of mental patients. Geneva: World Health Organisation.

World Health Organisation (1980). International classification of impairments, disabilities, and handicaps. Geneva: WHO.

World Health Organisation (2001). International classification of functioning, disability, and health. Geneva: World Health Organisation.

Worth, A. (2002). Health and Social Care assessment in action. In B. Blytheway, V. Bacigalupo, J. Bornat, J. Johnson & S. Spurr (eds.), Understanding Care, Welfare, and Community–a reader (pp. 321-329). London and New York: Routledge.

Index

Abstinence, as drug abuse treatment
policy, 122-123
Abuse, as psychosis risk factor,
219,220,221
Adaptation, environmental, 210
Addams, Jane, 11
Agency for Healthcare Research and
Quality, 81-82,85
AIDS patients. *See* HIV/AIDS patients
Alcohol
as legal drug, 121
as recreational drug, 119,120
Alcohol abuse, as physiological
dependence, 122
American Hospital Association, 11
American Medical Association,
Section on Hospitals, 12
Americans With Disabilities Act
(ADA), 50-52
Amphetamine abuse, in the United
Kingdom, 119
Animals, 210
Anti-sepsis, 14
Anxiety
in drug abusers, 128
reactivity-related, 219-220
social stressors-related, 221
Argyris, Chris, 44
Asthma, 222
Australia Institute of Health and
Welfare, 82
Australian National Health
Information Management
Group Working Party on
Health Outcomes Priorities,
79
Australia's Health 2000, 81
Autonomy, 210
Ayurveda medicine, 98

Balanced scorecards, 48
Bellevue Hospital, 9
Benzodiazepine abuse, as
physiological dependence,
122
Bereavement counseling, 180,186,187
Blair, Tony, 125
Boston, immigrant population of, 13
Boston Children's Aid Society, 9
Boston School for Social Work, 9,11
Botswana, home-based care for
HIV/AIDS patients in,
175-193
bereavement counseling component
of, 180
client and caregiver dissatisfaction
with, 180-183
concept of, 177-183
hospice care as alternative to,
183-191
bereavement counseling in,
186,187
characteristics of, 184-186
children's services in, 186,
187-188,189
family villages as, 186,188-189
Gaborone Declaration regarding,
191
guidelines for, 183-184
halfway houses as, 188
North East District
Multi-Sectoral AIDS
Committee program, 187-188
implications for HIV/AIDS-related
discrimination, 178-179
in Kweneng District, 180-183
objectives of, 177
obstacles to utilization of, 181,183

Printed and bound by CPI Group (UK) Ltd, Croydon, CR0 4YY

24/10/2024

01778906-0001